The Intermittent Fasting for Women Over 50

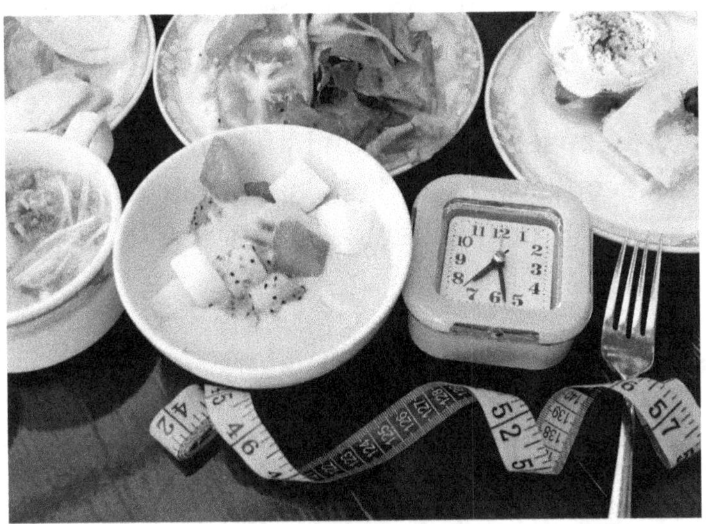

A Comprehensive, Step-by-Step Manual for Shedding Pounds, Restoring Your Body, and Incinerating Fat In <u>30 days</u>.

Dr.Rebecca J. Reynolds

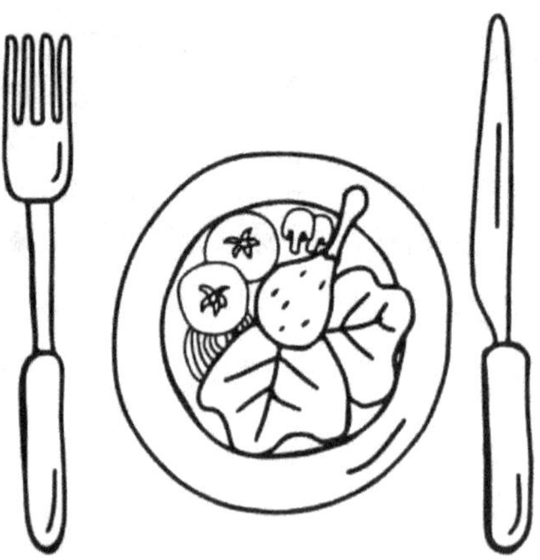

Table Of Content

INTRODUCTION

Fifty. A milestone. A number whispered across the media, paired with images of airbrushed models and unattainable expectations. But what if your fifties weren't about defying time, but about reclaiming your body and rewriting the narrative?

This isn't another faddy diet promising overnight miracles. *This is Intermittent Fasting for Women Over 50: A Comprehensive, Step-by-Step Manual for Shedding Pounds, Restoring Your Body, and Incinerating Fat In 30 Days.*– your guide to harnessing the power of time to transform your health and rediscover your vibrant self.

Forget crash diets and calorie counting. Forget starving yourself or grueling workouts that leave you aching. This book is about working smarter, not harder. It's about aligning your natural rhythms with a science-backed eating strategy that finally works for your changing body.

Here's a peek at what awaits you:

- **Unmasking the Myth of Menopause Weight:** We'll bust the stereotypes and delve into the hormonal shifts that make traditional diets ineffective for women over 50.
- **Your Personalized Fasting Map:** Discover the diverse range of intermittent fasting schedules and find the perfect fit for your lifestyle and preferences.
- **Nourishing Your Body, Not Depriving It:**Learn how to eat delicious, satisfying meals within your eating window, ensuring you reach your nutritional goals and ditch the hangry monster.
- **Beyond the Scale: Unveiling the Hidden Benefits:** We'll explore the wealth of health advantages beyond weight loss,from boosted energy and mental clarity to improved sleep and a stronger immune system.
- **Step-by-Step Implementation and Troubleshooting:** This is your action plan,complete with practical tips, expert advice,and solutions to overcome common challenges.

This book is more than just a guide; it's a supportive companion on your journey to reclaiming your health and confidence. We'll celebrate your victories, tackle setbacks together, and empower you to become the master of your own metabolism.

Are you ready to turn back the clock, not on your age, but on your limitations? Let's rewrite the narrative and make your fifties the decade you thrive, radiate, and incinerate fat for good. Dive into Intermittent Fasting for Women Over 50 and step into your healthiest, most vibrant self.

It's not just about shedding pounds, it's about shedding decades of doubt and igniting a new era of well-being. Your time is now.

A frequently asked query

1. Q:What is intermittent fasting (IF)?
   A: Intermittent fasting is an eating pattern that cycles between periods of eating and fasting.

2. Q: How does IF work?
   A:IF works by changing when you eat, allowing the body to utilize stored fat for energy during fasting periods.

3. Q:Are there different methods of intermittent fasting?
   A:Yes, popular methods include the 16/8 method, 5:2 diet, and the eat-stop-eat approach.

4. Q:Can I drink water during fasting periods?
   A:Yes, staying hydrated with water, tea, or black coffee is encouraged during fasting.

5. Q: Does intermittent fasting help with weight loss?

A: Yes, IF can aid weight loss by reducing calorie intake and promoting fat burning.

6. Q: What are the potential health benefits of IF?
A:Improved insulin sensitivity, cellular repair, and metabolic health are some reported benefits.

7. Q:Is IF suitable for everyone?
A: It may not be suitable for pregnant women, individuals with certain health conditions, or those with a history of eating disorders.

8. Q:Can I exercise during fasting periods?
A:Yes, moderate exercise is generally safe during fasting and may enhance the benefits.

9. Q:How long does it take to see results with intermittent fasting?
A:Results vary, but many people notice changes in a few weeks to a few months.

10. Q:Can I eat anything during the eating window?

A: While there's flexibility, focusing on nutrient-dense foods is recommended for overall health.

11. Q: Will intermittent fasting slow down my metabolism?
   A:IF may actually boost metabolism by promoting fat loss and preserving lean muscle mass.

12. Q: Should I consult a doctor before starting intermittent fasting?
   A: It's advisable, especially if you have underlying health conditions or are on medications.

13. Q:Does IF impact muscle mass?
   A: IF, when combined with resistance training, can help preserve or even build muscle.

14. Q:Can I do intermittent fasting every day?
   A:Yes, it can be done daily or intermittently based on individual preferences.

15. Q: Does IF have an impact on hormones?

A:Yes, IF can influence hormones like insulin, ghrelin, and norepinephrine, contributing to its effects.

16. Q:Can I do intermittent fasting while breastfeeding?
A: It's recommended to consult a healthcare professional, as nutritional needs may differ.

17. Q: Can IF improve mental clarity and focus?
A:Some individuals report improved cognitive function during fasting periods.

18. Q:What should I eat during the eating window?
A:Focus on a balanced diet with adequate protein, healthy fats, and a variety of fruits and vegetables.

19. Q:Can IF prevent or manage type 2 diabetes?
A:IF may improve insulin sensitivity and help manage blood sugar levels.

20. Q: Will intermittent fasting make me feel fatigued?

   A:Initially, some people may experience fatigue, but it often improves as the body adjusts.

21. Q: Can I have snacks during the fasting window?

   A: It's generally advised to avoid calorie-containing snacks, as they can break the fast.

22. Q:Does IF affect sleep patterns?

   A: It varies, but some people report improved sleep quality with IF.

23. Q: Can I drink alcohol during intermittent fasting?

   A:Alcohol can break the fast, so it's best to consume it while eating.

24. Q:How long should the fasting period be?

   A:The fasting period can range from 12 to 20 hours, depending on the chosen method.

25. Q: Can IF help reduce inflammation?

A:Some studies suggest that IF may have anti-inflammatory effects.

26. Q:Will intermittent fasting cause muscle loss?
A:When combined with proper nutrition and exercise, IF can help preserve muscle mass.

27. Q: Can I do intermittent fasting if I have a physically demanding job?
A: Yes, adjustments can be made to match fasting periods with rest or less active work hours.

28. Q: Is it normal to feel hungry during fasting periods?
A:Yes, initial hunger is common, but it often diminishes as the body adapts to the new eating pattern.

29. Q:Can intermittent fasting be done long-term?
A:Many people find it sustainable as a long-term lifestyle choice.

30. Q: Are there potential side effects of intermittent fasting?

A: Side effects may include initial hunger, irritability, or changes in sleep patterns, but they often improve over time.

Fundamentals of Intermittent fasting.

In essence, fasting involves refraining from food consumption, constituting a purposeful act of withholding nourishment from the body for more than six hours. Conversely, intermittent fasting emerges as a nutritional strategy encompassing prolonged intervals of fasting over several days, interspersed with periods allowing food intake, albeit with some prudent considerations. This approach need not be a daily commitment, as individuals can tailor it to align with their specific objectives and lifestyles.

During the feeding windows, a diverse range of foods can be consumed, emphasizing low-calorie options such as meat, fish, eggs, while moderating the intake of simple sugars and opting for items with a low glycemic index. Whole grains, legumes, dried and fresh fruits, and healthy fats are also encouraged. One variant of intermittent fasting involves cyclic fasting patterns to curtail overall daily caloric intake.

The primary objective is to redirect the body's focus away from constant digestion. This temporal absence of food in the stomach triggers metabolic changes, allowing the body to prioritize recovery and maintenance processes. While some may perceive fasting as detrimental, scientific research, as reported by Healthline, asserts its positive impact on both the mind and body. Fasting not only aids in effortless weight loss by reducing overall calorie intake but also enhances metabolic function. It fosters self-discipline, combats unhealthy eating habits, and serves as an umbrella term encompassing various voluntary fasting forms.

Intermittent fasting encompasses three main approaches to food abstinence: alternate-day fasting, daily restrictions, and periodic fasting. While methods may differ, the overarching goal remains consistent—cultivating a healthier metabolism, achieving an optimal body weight, and promoting an active lifestyle. The American Heart Association (AHA) has delved into intermittent fasting, attributing benefits such as countering insulin resistance, addressing cardio-metabolic diseases, and facilitating weight loss. However, questions persist about the sustainability of this health-effective method.

The 2019 research paper, "Effects of intermittent fasting on health, aging, and disease," further supports intermittent fasting's efficacy against insulin resistance, inflammation, hypertension, obesity, and dyslipidemia. Nevertheless, ongoing exploration is crucial, with a focus on reconciling traditional fasting practices deeply ingrained in various religions, from Buddhism to Jainism, Orthodox Christianity, Hinduism, and Islam, with the contemporary era of science and technology. The evolution of these age-old practices in the context of modern research underscores the nuanced exploration of their relevance in promoting holistic well-being.

The Mechanisms Underpinning Intermittent Fasting

Intermittent fasting has a variety of biological effects, including cellular proliferation, gene expression, and body expansion. To comprehend the science underlying the mechanisms of intermittent fasting, one must study the roles played by insulin, human growth hormones, cellular repair, and gene expression. Insulin levels are then reduced by intermittent fasting, which first decreases glucose levels. This reduction in insulin aids in the body's fat burning, progressively reducing obesity and associated illnesses. Insulin resistance and diabetes are also avoided by maintaining controlled insulin levels. Conversely, periodic fasting increases the amount of human growth hormones five times or more. HGH production is elevated, which promotes rapid muscular growth and fat burning.

The body begins the process of self-healing at the cellular level when under fasting, eliminating undesirable, non-functional cells and detritus in the process. This has a purifying impact that feeds the body either directly or indirectly and permits it to develop in an environment with less oxidative stress. Similarly, fasting even modifies the expression of certain genes in the human body. The coding and decoding of gene expression determines how a cell behaves; transcription that proceeds normally in a healthy environment naturally contributes to cell lifespan, and fasting guarantees uninterrupted transcription. Thus, by fortifying bodily cells, intermittent fasting combats aging, cancer, and strengthens the immune system.

How It Operates

Eating is an essential need that we fulfill continuously from birth. We introduce food into our bodies every day. At the point when we eat, the digestion actuates itself to begin the stomach related process. This cycle utilizes an enormous measure of energy. The more food we present, the more the body should attempt to utilize it. Assuming the food is presented and to an extreme, or excessively brimming with sugars and fats the work that the stomach related framework should support but more prominent.

At the point when we are quick, nonetheless, we stop this cycle and this energy apportioning. The saved energy is in this manner redirected to other metabolic cycles, basically of a helpful kind.

By removing toxins through its emunctory organs, the body that is not engaged in food digestion can better devote itself to purification. These enormous inner cleanings clearly have positive repercussions on the condition of wellbeing of organs and tissues. The life form is detoxified and rejuvenated.

American scientists at Yale's Institute of Medication featured how throughout the break from food, our creature delivers a substance fit for quenching persistent irritation. It is known as the β-hydroxybutyrate (BHB) and its proficient transform falls into a perplexing arrangement of proteins that guide the fiery reaction in numerous pathologies, including a few immune system illnesses. A decent outcome recommends how later on remedial fasting can be utilized in the early treatment of numerous fiery based illnesses.

Irregular fasting is a device that can assist us with enacting the cycles portrayed above and face a genuine quick. It works between exchanging times of eating and fasting, as a matter of fact. It is a considerably more adaptable methodology, as there are numerous choices to browse as indicated by body type, size, weight objectives, and wholesome necessities.

The human body works like a synchronized machine that calls for adequate investment for self-recuperation and fix. At the point when we continually eat garbage and undesirable food or too high an amount of food without the thought of our caloric requirements, it prompts heftiness and poisonous development in the body. For that reason fasting comes as a characteristic method for detoxifying the body and giving it sufficient opportunity to use its fat stores.

Anything that the human body consumes is at last broken into glucose, which is subsequently used by the cells in glycolysis to deliver energy. As the blood glucose level ascents, insulin is created to bring down the levels and permit the liver to do Again Lipogenesis, the cycle in which the overabundant glucose is transformed into glycogen and at last put away into fat, bringing about stoutness. By deliberately causing energy deprivation, intermittent fasting appears to reverse this process by breaking down the existing fat.

Discontinuous fasting manages lipolysis; however it is a characteristic body process, it must be started when the blood glucose levels drop to an adequately depressed spot. That point can be accomplished through fasting and working out. At the point when an individual removes the outside glucose supply for a few

hours, the body changes to lipolysis. This course of breaking the fats additionally delivers other side-effects like ketones which are fit for decreasing the oxidative pressure of the body and help in its detoxification.

Mark Mattson, a neuroscientist from Johns Hopkins Medication College, has read up irregular fasting for nearly 25 years of his vocation. He spread out the functions of irregular fasting by explaining its clinical application and the science behind it. As indicated by him, discontinuous fasting should be picked for a sound way of life.

While examining the use of this dietary methodology, it is basic to comprehend how discontinuous fasting stands apart from easygoing slimming down rehearses. It's more than just not eating at all. What is eaten in this dietary way of life is similarly significant as the actual fasting. It doesn't bring about hunger; rather, it advances smart dieting alongside the quick. Irregular fasting is partitioned into two distinct states that follow each other. The cycle begins with the "FED" state, which is trailed by a "Fasting" state. The method of intermittent fasting is used to determine the duration of the fasting state and the frequency of the FED state. The last option is portrayed by high blood glucose levels, though during the fasting state the body goes through a continuous decrease in glucose levels. This decrease in glucose flags the pancreas and the cerebrum to meet the body's energy needs by handling the accessible fat particles. In any case, on the off chance that the fasting state is trailed by a Took care of state in which an individual gorges food rich in carbs and fats, it will end up being more risky for their wellbeing. As a result, a healthy diet must accompany the fasting period.

Benefits of Intermittent Fasting on Health

You must have been aware up until this point that intermittent fasting is merely switching between eating and fasting. Eating is finished in cycles or explicit periods and fasting is not very far behind. There are various advantages of discontinuous fasting.

Periodic Loss of Weight:

Fasting involves alternating between eating and fasting intervals. Naturally, fasting lowers your caloric intake and aids in the maintenance of your weight reduction. It also keeps you from overindulging in food. Your body turns food into fat and glucose whenever you eat it. It stores the fat for later use and consumes this glucose right away. Your body begins to draw on its internal fat reserves for energy when you miss a few meals. Additionally, the majority of the fat you lose comes from your abdomen. This diet is ideal for those who wish to have a flat tummy.

Addresses Diabetes:

Even in isolation, diabetes poses a serious risk. Additionally, it serves as a key marker for the rise in risk factors associated with a number of cardiovascular illnesses, including strokes and heart attacks. Diabetes is brought on by a dangerously high blood glucose level and insufficient insulin to handle the glucose. Controlling the body's insulin levels becomes challenging when the body rejects insulin. Diabetes can be managed and insulin sensitivity is decreased with intermittent fasting.

slumber:

One of the primary reasons for obesity is sleep deprivation. Your body's internal fat-burning system fails when it doesn't get enough sleep. Your sleep cycle is regulated by intermittent fasting, which helps your body burn fat efficiently. Numerous physiological advantages of a healthy sleep cycle include increased energy and mood.

Adaptation to Illnesses

Occasionally fasting aids in the development and renewal of cells. The human body contains an internal system that aids in the mending of damaged cells. Did you know that? A periodic fast aids in the activation of this process. It enhances the body's cells' general ability to function. As a result, it immediately contributes to strengthening your body's defenses against sickness and disease by making it more resistant to them.

A Healthy Heart

Intermittent Fasting assists in weight loss, and weight loss improves your cardiovascular health. A buildup of plaque in blood vessels is known as atherosclerosis. This is the primary cause of various cardiovascular diseases. The endothelium is the thin lining of blood vessels, and any dysfunction in it results in atherosclerosis. Obesity is the primary problem that plagues humanity and is also the main reason for the increase of plaque deposits in the blood vessels. Stress and inflammation also increase the severity of this problem. Intermittent Fasting tackles the buildup of fat and helps tackle obesity. So, all you need to do is follow the simple protocols of Intermittent Fasting to improve your overall health.

A Healthy Gut:

There are several millions of microorganisms present in your digestive system. These microorganisms help improve the overall functioning of your digestive system and are known as the gut microbiome. Intermittent Fasting enhances the health of these microbiomes and improves your digestive health. A healthy digestive system helps in better absorption of food and improves the functioning of your stomach.

Reduces Inflammation:

Whenever your body feels there is an internal problem, its natural defense is inflammation. It doesn't mean that all forms of inflammation are desirable. Inflammation can cause several serious health conditions like arthritis, atherosclerosis, and other neurodegenerative disorders.

Any inflammation of this nature is known as chronic inflammation and is quite painful. Chronic inflammation can restrict your body's movements too.

Encourages Cell Replacement:

Your body's cells begin the process of eliminating waste when you fast. Waste disposal, also referred to as autophagy, is the process by which all defective cells and proteins are broken down. Autophagy provides defense against cancer and a number of degenerative illnesses, including Alzheimer's. You dislike having a lot of trash around your house, don't you? In a similar vein, your body shouldn't retain any needless poisons. The body uses autophagy as a means of eliminating everything unnecessary.

Higher Concentration and Brain Power:

When subjected to food scarcity for a long time, mammals, including humans, will start to experience a decrease in their organ size. One of these organs is the brain. While some organs return to their original size over time, others may be impacted over the long term.

The brain handles the basic cognitive function of the body. In order to function properly and get the needed nutrients, it needs to return to its original size. However, if the brain becomes too foggy, getting the needed food nutrients will be pretty difficult, which might lead to malnutrition and even be fatal. However, during a shorter period of food scarcity, the brain becomes hyperactive in its search for food as a mechanism for survival.

Excessive availability of food and eating altogether makes us mentally dull. Reflect on a time when you were completely satisfied after a big meal. After eating a massive plate of food, you will likely go into a "food coma" and curl up and sleep, or maybe just watch your favorite TV show on Netflix rather than get the motivation to go achieve your goals. Without a doubt, satisfaction from food makes man naturally lose the drive to pursue his goals, which ultimately leads to dulling the brain. With this in mind, know that when you fast, your cognitive abilities are quickened. This improves your mental keenness, allowing you to achieve your health- related goals as opposed to excessively feeding.

It should be established here that there is no scientific research to support the notion that intermittent fasting alters mental alertness negatively. Fasting will not affect your cognitive function, such as moods, mental alertness, reaction time, intention, and sleep in any bad way. On the contrary, these things get boosted during fasting.

Promotes Autophagy and Protects Neurons:

This is one of the many wonderful benefits of intermittent fasting, which many people should look forward to. Fasting is amazing in that it keeps the brain's cells from degeneration. This is because fasting prevents neural death.

Besides, fasting also triggers the process of autophagy in the brain— autophagy is the process in which the body gets rid of damaged body cells and brings out new ones. When the body is full of healthy, active, and improved cells, it is strong and well-equipped to combat any diseases that might want to attack.

Autophagy significantly lowers the likelihood of viral infection and intracellular parasite duplication. As a result, intracellular pathogens like cancer cells are drastically reduced. In addition, aberrant development, inflammation, and toxicity are prevented from harming brain and other bodily tissue cells.

Diminished Chance of Depression:

There is a rise in the neurotransmitter "neurotrophic factor" when there is an intermittent fast. A deficiency of this brain-derived substance in the body leads to serious problems like depression and other mood disorders. Thus, intermittent fasting is very beneficial for elevating mood and mental clarity, both of which decrease the likelihood of developing these diseases.

Fasting improves brain health through a few metabolic processes that are activated. This explains why there is a decrease in oxidative stress, blood sugar, and inflammation in those who follow intermittent fasting.

Additionally, there are signs that intermittent fasting can maintain the brain's defenses against stroke risk.

Increases Immune Regulation

During a fast, the body's primary goal is to maintain a healthy immune system. To this end we empower drinking an enormous amount of water during the time of the irregular quick, and a while later too. Water can be brightened up with other detox specialists that eliminate poisons from the stomach related framework and decrease the quantity of undesirable stomach microorganisms. Have at the top of the priority list that the quantity of stomach organisms present in the gastrointestinal parcel is straightforwardly connected with the resistant framework's capability.

The body's level of inflammatory cytokines is determined by intermittent fasting. As a result, it aids in immune system regulation. In the body, we have two huge cytokines that cause irritation in the body: Both tumor necrosis factor alpha and interleukin-6 These inflammatory pro-inflammatory cytokines are less likely to be released when people fast.

Lessens the Gamble of Persistent Sickness:

Individuals living with persistent immune system illnesses like Crohn's infection, colitis, rheumatoid joint inflammation, and fundamental lupus will see amazing improvement with irregular fasting. The thought is straightforward. These individuals experience a slower rate of an extreme inflammatory process in their bodies when they fast. With this, they have an optimal insusceptible capability.

For example, disease cells have somewhere in the range of ten and seventy additional insulin receptors as opposed to sound body cells. This occurs because sugar is broken down into fuel. With discontinuous fasting, disease cells are famished from sugar consumption. This conditions the cells for harm through free extremists.

Further develops Hereditary Fix Instruments

The propensity of the body to live longer increments when it doesn't get sufficient food. This is on the grounds that, with irregular fasting, there is fix and recovery of cells that come about by means of a maintenance component in the body. This is reasonable, as the energy expected for cell fix is lesser when contrasted with what is fundamental for cell creation or division.

Consequently, during the time of irregular fasting, cell division, and creation in the body becomes decreased. This is a fundamental cycle, crucial particularly for the recuperating of dangerous cells, which flourish because of unusual cell division.

In the body, the human development chemical (HGH) deals with the course of cell fix. A human development chemical gets out changes digestion that cause tissue fix and fat consuming. In this way, when we quick, the body can focus more on fixing body tissues with amino acids and compounds. This reestablishes tissue collagen and furthermore sets off an improvement in bones, tendons, ligaments, and general muscle capability in the body.

Decrease the Probability of Creating Malignant growth

Finally, investigations have discovered that irregular fasting can decrease your probability of creating disease and assist with making treatment more effective. As you know, irregular fasting can assist with treating oxidative pressure and cell harm, the two of which cause disease. By lessening this harm, you can accordingly diminish your gamble of creating malignant growth later on.

Yet, that isn't all. While human examinations actually should be directed, a concentrate on mice found that while rehearsing momentary fasting, chemotherapy therapy moves to the next level in focusing on and treating both bosom malignant growth and skin disease. Not in the least did the actual chemotherapy become more viable, however the mice's safe frameworks likewise were better ready to fend off the carcinogenic cells and developments, which is fundamental as chemotherapy is notable for lessening an individual's resistant framework radically.

The Best Method During Menopause

Menopause is perhaps the most convoluted work in a lady's life. At the point when our bodies start to change and significant normal advances happen that are time and again adversely impacted, while it is vital to figure out how to change our dietary patterns and eating designs properly. In point of fact, it frequently occurs that a woman is not prepared for this new condition and experiences it with a sense of defeat as an unavoidable sign of time travel. This feeling of prostration, on the other hand, turns out to be excessively intrusive and involves numerous parts of the stomach.

It is hence vital to resist the urge to panic when there are messages about the main indications of progress in our human body, to avert the beginning of menopause for the right reason and to limit the adverse consequences of misery, particularly in the good 'ol days. In any event, during this troublesome progress, designated nourishment can be exceptionally useful.

What A Menopausal Woman's Body Goes Through

It should be said that a fair eating routine doesn't deliver significant weight variances. This will undoubtedly be a factor that helps women who are going through menopause, but it is not enough to present with typical symptoms that can be categorized based on the time period. Truth be told, we can recognize the perimenopausal stage, which influences somewhere in the range of 45 and 50 years, and is physiologically viable with an uncommon decrease in the creation of the chemical estrogen (liable for the monthly cycle, which really begins sporadically). A number of complex and highly subjective endocrine changes occur during this time.

When a person goes through the actual menopause, the amount of estrogen hormone produced decreases even more, and the range of symptoms increases. This causes a lot of the hormone, like the catecholamine adrenaline class. The consequence of these progressions is a risky intensity wave, expanded perspiring, and the presence of tachycardia, which can be pretty extreme.

Notwithstanding, the progressions likewise influence the female genital organs, with the volume of the bosoms, uterus and ovaries diminishing. Vaginal dryness rises as a result of the decreased activity of the mucous membranes. There may likewise be changes in bone equilibrium, with diminished calcium consumption and expanded activation to the detriment of the skeletal framework. Along these lines, there is an absence of persistent bone development, and on the other hand, disintegration starts, which is an inclination for osteoporosis.

Despite the fact that menopause causes significant changes that extraordinarily change a lady's body and soul, digestion is quite possibly horrible. As a matter of fact, during menopause, the retention and collection of sugars and fatty substances changes and it is not difficult to expand a few clinical qualities, for example, cholesterol and fatty oils, which lead to hypertension or arteriosclerosis. Furthermore, numerous ladies frequently grumble of upsetting circulatory problems and nearby edema, particularly in the stomach. It additionally makes weight gain simpler, despite the fact that you haven't changed your dietary patterns.

The Optimal Menopausal Diet

In situations where issues connected with the appearance of menopause become challenging to make due, medication or regular treatment under clinical watch might be important. The commitment given by a right eating regimen as of now can be significant, as a matter of fact, given the significant factors that become an integral factor, it is important to alter our food normal, both all together not to be shocked by this large number of changes, and to adjust in the most potential regular manner.

The issue of fat gathering in the stomach region is constantly brought about by the drop-in estrogen. As a matter of fact, they are likewise liable for the exemplary hourglass state of most ladies, which comprises in keeping fat fundamentally on the hips, which starts to fall flat with menopause. Thus, we go from a gynoid condition to an android one, with a fat increment limited on the gut. Furthermore, the metabolic pace of removal is diminished, and that implies that regardless of whether you change your eating regimen and eat similar amounts of food as you generally have, you could encounter weight gain, which will be more set apart within the sight of vices or unpredictable eating routine.

Additionally, digestion takes longer and the function of the intestines becomes more complicated. Swelling and the development of previously unnoticed intolerances and digestive disorders are both exacerbated by this. Consequently, the starting will be more risky and hard to oversee during this period. The appropriation of supplements should be unique: diminishing how much low starch, which is constantly avoided the chance to

be filtered, evades the pinnacle of insulin and simultaneously keeps up with stable glucose.
Moreover, it will be important to build the amount of both creature and vegetable proteins somewhat; Select healthy fats, favor seeds and extra-virgin olive oil, and strictly limit saturated fatty acids (those derived from animals like lard, lard, and so on). This is to attempt to build the extent of cell reinforcements taken, which will assist with checking the impact of free revolutionaries, whose fixation starts to increment during this period. It will be important to favor food sources rich in phytoestrogens, which will assist with controlling the conditions of pressure to which the body is oppressed and which will lean toward, in some measure to a limited extent, the in general estrogenic equilibrium.

These particles are isolated into three principal gatherings and the food sources that contain them ought to never be absent on our tables: isoflavones, which are mostly found in legumes like soy and red clover; lignans, of which flax seeds and sleek seeds, as a general rule, are especially rich; cumestani, found in sunflower seeds, beans and fledglings. Calcium supplementation will be essential through cheeses like parmesan; egg yolks, yogurt, certain vegetables like rocket, Brussels sprouts, broccoli, spinach, and asparagus, legumes; dried natural products like nuts, almonds or dried grapes.

Magnificent extra propensities that will assist with recapturing prosperity might be: limiting sweets to occasional occasions and drastically reducing sugar intake (for example, By opting for herbal tea instead of sugary beverages and acquiring a taste for its natural flavors.); figuring out how to portion liquor a great deal (keeping away from spirits, mixers and aperitif drinks) and pick just a single glass of good wine when you are in organization, this since it will in general increment instinctive fat which is unequivocally the thing will settle at the level stomach. Obviously, even by eating heaps of organic product, arriving at a high starch quantity as in a conventional diet is troublesome. Nonetheless, a dietary plan can be valuable to have a more exact sign of how to disperse the food sources. Clearly, one's eating routine should be organized in an individual manner, in light of explicit metabolic necessities and one's way of life.

Choosing the Best Intermittent Fasting Method for Men Over 50 (Andropause)

situations where the challenges associated with aging become prominent for men over 50, a strategic dietary approach, such as intermittent fasting, can be pivotal. While medication and clinical supervision might be necessary, a well-structured eating regimen becomes crucial to adapt to the changes that accompany this phase of life.

One common issue faced by men over 50 is the tendency for fat accumulation in the abdominal region. The decline in certain hormones, including testosterone, can contribute to a shift in body composition. Unlike women experiencing menopause, men may encounter challenges related to maintaining a lean physique. The metabolic rate decreases, and the intricacies of digestive functions increase, making weight management more complex, especially when faced with irregular eating patterns.

Intermittent fasting offers a potential solution by optimizing the timing of food consumption. The extended periods of fasting can promote fat utilization for energy, addressing the challenges associated with abdominal fat accumulation. However, considering the metabolic changes during this phase, men should approach intermittent fasting with thoughtful considerations.

The slowing of metabolism and increased complexity of digestive functions can make the initiation of intermittent fasting more challenging for men over 50. Starting gradually, with shorter fasting windows and gradually extending them, allows the body to adapt more comfortably. Intermittent fasting may also help reduce the risk of insulin spikes, contributing to more stable glucose levels, an important consideration for overall health in this age group.

In addition to adjusting the fasting periods, modifying nutrient intake becomes crucial. Emphasizing a balanced distribution of macronutrients is essential. Slightly increasing both animal and plant-based proteins is advisable. Opting for healthy fats, such as those found in seeds and extra-virgin olive oil, while strictly limiting saturated fatty acids from animal sources, aligns with the goal of supporting overall health.

Furthermore, incorporating foods rich in antioxidants is vital to combat the increasing concentration of free radicals associated with aging. A focus on phytoestrogen-rich foods may not be as relevant for men, but prioritizing antioxidants from various sources can still be beneficial. These include fruits, vegetables, nuts, and seeds.

Calcium supplementation remains crucial for bone health, and sources like dairy products, egg yolks, and certain vegetables should be included. Integrating intermittent fasting into a dietary plan for men over 50 requires careful consideration of individual metabolic needs and lifestyle, ensuring it aligns with their overall well-being.

Additional positive habits that contribute to well-being include limiting sweets to occasional treats, reducing alcohol intake, and choosing moderate wine consumption during social occasions. As with any dietary plan, individualization is key, taking into account specific metabolic requirements and lifestyle preferences.

Intermittent fasting can be a valuable approach for men over 50 to address the challenges associated with aging. By gradually incorporating fasting windows, adjusting nutrient intake, and prioritizing a well-balanced diet, men can leverage intermittent fasting as a tool for maintaining a healthy weight and overall well-being during this phase of life.

Advice and Techniques For All

Before you start fasting, there are things that you believe you should do to set yourself up. It could be troublesome intellectually and actually, particularly assuming you are new to fasting. Your outlook will turn out to be vital as you are fasting, particularly the more you quick at one time.

Detoxify your Body

Your body is a brilliant piece of inventive sorcery that was worked to work for the whole length of your life on the planet. It comprises various complex frameworks, every one of which plays an essential part to play in supporting your life. The negative effects on the body as a whole can be devastating if any of these systems are compromised in any way.

As you age, irritation frequently turns into a test. Begin by considering the kind of food you are presently eating that might be causing irritation. Plan your eating routine to reject whatever number of these food sources as could be expected under the circumstances:

- Refined sugar: This is tracked down in cakes, treats, sugar, and pastries.
- Refined starches: This is tracked down in bread, pasta, baked goods, and treats.
- Handled meats: Some are ham, salami, bacon, and jerky
- Food varieties with MSG: A few food varieties are moment noodles, moment crush, and so on.
- Fake trans-fats: This can be tracked down in specific margarine, French fries, quick food varieties, microwave popcorn, and so on.
- Alcohol.

- Vegetable and seed oils: Soy and sunflower seed oil are two examples.

Incorporate a wide assortment of calming food varieties like broccoli, new vegetables, natural products, lean meat, fish, and bunches of water.

Guarantee You Are Fasting in a Sound Manner

With regards to fasting, it is essential to guarantee that you approach it such that it will be advantageous for your wellbeing, and that won't cause more damage than great.

You, first and foremost, need to keep up with adaptability with yourself and your body while fasting. On the off chance that you are not feeling good as you are attempting to quick, don't hesitate for even a moment to eat a modest quantity on your quick days. This is particularly obvious toward the start when you initially bring fasting into your eating regimen. Assuming you attempt a water quick for instance, and you feel tipsy and frail, you might conclude that you need to rather attempt an irregular fasting technique like 5:2 which would permit you to eat on your quick days, however in an extraordinarily confined sum.

Acquire Legitimate Nourishment and Rest

Dozing is a fundamental piece of human existence, and getting how much rest a body needs to run well will help you in irregular fasting, keeping you dynamic.

Assuming you're endeavoring 24-hour water quick, ensure that the last feast of your day is eaten well before sleep time. In the hour leading up to bedtime, consume something nutritious that isn't overly loaded with fat or carbohydrates and drink a lot of water so that when hunger strikes, your body has enough nutrients to last at least three or four hours.

Make sure to eat a lot of fruits when they are in season and schedule breaks for food and rest if you are doing a multi-day fast or one where you will be working or walking outside. Take some time to sit down and eat something if you feel lightheaded or weak from hunger so you don't have to stop the fast for a meal. Fasting ought to never be debilitating or awkward, so verify that you're

getting enough of what your body needs during the day so that it's not difficult to proceed.

Rolling out huge improvements in your eating routine or endeavoring things like fasting too early prior to taking some time off can be extremely distressing and negative to your general wellbeing, so don't rush it. Instead of making drastic changes right away, focus on eating healthier foods over time.

While you're eating each and every other day, don't fear attempting new food varieties or planning dinners in various ways. Break free from the same old foods you've been eating for years. You deserve it. Go ahead and move toward your food arranging uniquely in contrast to you regularly would, and remember to appreciate it!

Include Some Physical Activity

If at all possible, try to get some physical activity in before starting your first fast so that your body is ready for what lies ahead. Regardless of whether you resolve during the week, you will be consuming undeniably a bigger number of calories than ordinary while fasting and it would be really smart to set up your body somehow or another.

Only a couple of moments every day are sufficient, in any case, and as you become acclimated to doing as such, you can build the length of your exercises until you feel at ideal wellbeing. Along these lines, when you do quick, your body encounters no deficiency of energy and can keep up its generally expected capabilities.

Strolling is a great type of activity for weight reduction that requires no extraordinary hardware or preparing. If you are accustomed to working out on weekends, you can also try doing some aerobic exercises.

With regards to the weight reduction advantages of fasting, there's no deficiency of data, and studies have demonstrated that a delayed time of fasting can prompt a huge weight reduction.

The main thing you'll require is a dehydrator and some food - indeed, you can in any case go through the most common way of fasting regardless of whether you're working! You simply have to ensure you generally have snacks with you so your body will not get too eager constantly. You will likewise have to know when you ought to hydrate, as well as what sorts of food sources you ought to and shouldn't eat.

Continuously make sure to have breakfast, nibble on protein-rich food sources over the course of the day, get a decent night's rest and hydrate. This is actually somewhat easy and will help you look thin as well as be sound. There are numerous ways for you to get in shape quickly, however the best strategy is through eating fewer carbs and practicing appropriately.

Increment Your Water Admission

Lack of hydration can go with fasting since a lot of our water consumption over the course of the day comes from the food we eat, similar to natural products or vegetables. Assuming you are feeling like you are got dried out while fasting (dry mouth, migraine), expanding your water intake is significant. You will likewise need to guarantee you hydrate each time you quick thereafter. The suggestion is around two liters each day, obviously, this relies upon your body size. In general, you should drink eight glasses of water, each about eight ounces in weight, to stay hydrated. However, if you are fasting, you should drink nine to thirteen glasses. This amounts to approximately two to three liters of water.

Focus on Your Body

On the off chance that you are feeling exceptionally unwell while you are fasting, it is vital to know when to quit fasting. It is ordinary to feel exhausted, hungry, and perhaps crabby when you are quick, however you might need to stop your quick on the off chance that you feel totally unwell. Keep the duration of your first few fasts short to ensure safety, and gradually increase it to the desired duration. Likewise, keep some food on you in the event that you really want to eat something because of low glucose or feeling unwell. Keep in mind that you are fasting for health and body care, so it shouldn't make you feel worse.

Keep away from Pressure

At the point when we start a new thing, particularly on the off chance that it is connected with our body, we really want to consider the conceivable pressure it might cause. Worrying about it could make it most horrendously terrible. Resist the urge to panic, do your thing, and don't worry. Recollect that fasting suggests not eating food varieties for quite a while. While fasting, be steady with yourself and do whatever it takes not to eat before the named time. It will ensure that you lose the best measure of weight and get the most advantages from discontinuous fasting in strong terms.

Increment Protein Admission

Guaranteeing that you eat sufficient protein while fasting will have various advantages for you. Protein takes more time to process, and that implies that the energy you get from protein will be longer enduring than the energy you get from different sources like starches which are spent rapidly. This will hold you back from having an energy "crash" like a sugar crash after you have rapidly spent the sugars you have ingested.

Select the Food sources You Eat Astutely

At the point when you in all actuality do break your fast or when you are eating limited quantities on fasting days, pick the food sources you eat carefully. You must properly prepare your body for the fast in order to maintain its health. As well as eating sufficient protein, you need to ensure that different food sources you eat are genuine, entire food varieties. Entire food varieties are those which are as near those tracked down in nature as could be expected. These are things like meats, vegetables, organic products, fish, eggs, and vegetables. This will give you each of the supplements you really want to remain solid. Eating inexpensive food and handled food varieties when you are not fasting will leave you feeling tired and without energy, particularly assuming you are fasting the following day or have abstained the other day.

Think about Supplementation

Enhancing might be exceptionally valuable and, surprisingly, important while fasting to keep up with and further develop wellbeing. A few fundamental supplements and minerals that your body would significantly profit from like Omega-3's or press might be hard to get in sufficient sums assuming you are fasting. Thus, enhancing them might help you as far as keeping you feeling great and enthusiastic, as well as keeping your cerebrum working to its maximum capacity. You can take explicit supplements on their own in pill structure or you can select a multivitamin that will incorporate the most fundamental nutrients as a whole and minerals for generally speaking great wellbeing. The nutrients remembered for a multivitamin will be those that are known to advance great by and large wellbeing and those that are generally gotten through a fair, entire food diet.

Abstain from Getting carried away First and foremost

Downplaying your activity levels while fasting is much of the time important as your body won't have as some promptly accessible sugars or starches to furnish you with the speedy energy required for an exercise. This is particularly significant on the off chance that you are starting a fasting routine interestingly. On the off chance that you are wanting to build your degrees of autophagy through a mix of fasting and exercise, hold on until your body has adjusted to your fasting routine prior to including the activity piece of the arrangement.

Find Something to Do When You Quick

It is said that an idle psyche is Satan's display area. At the point when you quick discontinuously and are not occupied, food will be the main thing at the forefront of your thoughts, convincing you to eat before the quick breaking time. You can start reading or do research on anything that interests you, pick up a new skill, or start a hobby.

What to Eat and What Not to Eat

No matter how you plan your intermittent fasting journey, you need to understand what you can and can't eat during your effort. If you will not eat solid food for only 24 hours, you need to know exactly what you can eat on fasting days. Likewise, it would be good to know what works best for your non-fasting days. Remember: just because it's a non-fast day doesn't mean it's a good idea to go out and enjoy a buffet. In this chapter, we'll help you make healthy food decisions about what to eat and what not to eat during intermittent fasting.

what to eat

Berry

Berries are healthy, delicious, and contain far fewer calories and sugar than you might think! Their sweet sweetness can liven up smoothies and make a delicious snack on its own without the help of something like cream or sugar.

cruciferous vegetables

Vegetables such as cabbage, Brussels sprouts, broccoli and cauliflower. They are a great addition to your diet because they are full of essential nutrients and fiber that your body loves and uses quickly!

Egg

Eggs are a great addition to your diet because they're high in protein, can go with anything, are easy to prepare, hold up well when boiled, and go with almost anything. It's a great source of protein for salads, but it's also great on its own.

FISH

White fish in particular is generally very lean, but some colorful fish such as salmon are full of protein, healthy fats and oils. It's good for brain and heart health, and you can make lots of delicious things with it.

Starch as healthy as a single potato (even the skin!)

Red potatoes, in particular, can be eaten even if you want to lose weight, because they help your body use carbohydrates for fuel, and their skin is full of minerals that your body loves. A few potatoes here and there can help your diet, but it's also good to feel like you're eating some unusual foods that you need to cut back on.

legume

Peas, beans and magical fruits. They're full of protein, and the starch they contain helps them stick to your ribs without paying for them later. They are delicious in soups, salads and any other meal of the day you want to fill up on. Adding beans to your diet will help food stay with you longer and make you feel more satisfied than you ever imagined.

NUTS

You've probably heard people say that a handful of almonds is a great snack. If you're like me, you might find it hard to believe. Nuts are rich in healthy fats that your body can use to overcome rough patches. It's not the most satisfying snack on its own, but try filling up a salad. If you want a little crunch or to make it a little more satisfying, try it with berries.

Probiotics Help Improve Gut Health

Feeling happier usually means better nutritional success and overall health!

Vegetables Rich in Healthy Fats

It may not seem modern or trendy, but avocados are a great example of a vegetable rich in healthy fats. Look for vegetables rich in fatty acids and fats. Adding these vegetables to your diet will help you feel less hungry.

Water

Whatever you decide to add or subtract from your regimen, make sure you stay hydrated. It promotes digestion and prevents you from feeling hungry or tired. Add electrolytes as needed and don't be shy about taking a bottle with you as you move from place to place. Stay hydrated!

Grains

Whole grains may be healthy and high in fiber, but you can also get these nutrients from other sources. The human diet does not require the consumption of grains. The truth has a few advantages in cereals, but in general it is usually powerful, clean and not compatible with ketone diets.

Some people are known as a diet for planned systems, diet versions and various courses. People following a specific ketogenic diet eat small amounts of high-carbohydrate foods, such as whole grains, 30 to 40 minutes before exercising.

starchy vegetables and legumes

Some vegetables are high in carbohydrates. These include potatoes, beans, sugar beets and corn. While these vegetables may have nutritional benefits, you can get the same nutrients from low-carb plant-based alternatives.

sweet fruits

Since most fruits are high in sugar, they are also high in carbohydrates. It is important to avoid many fruits. The exception is that you can eat berries, lemons, and limes in moderation. Some people occasionally snack on small pieces of melon, but be careful with your portion size as it can add up quickly!

Milk and low-fat dairy products

Unfortunately, because you can enjoy dairy products like cheese on a ketogenic diet, milk contains more carbohydrates than cheese. One glass of 2% milk contains 12 carbohydrates, which is half of your daily total. Instead,Choose low-carb, dairy-free milk alternatives such as almond, coconut or soy milk.

Consider using low-fat cheese instead of full-fat cheese to reduce your saturated fat intake. This is because cheese is made from low-fat dairy products and is naturally higher in carbohydrates, lowering your daily net carb total.

Alcohol

Alcohol is generally discouraged on the ketogenic diet. That's because your body can't burn calories while your liver is trying to process the alcohol.

Many people find that they get drunk faster and experience severe hangovers when they are in ketosis. Plus, alcohol adds unnecessary calories and carbohydrates to your diet. The worst beers to choose from are margaritas, pina coladas, sangrias, bloody marys, whiskey sours, cosmopolitans, and regular beers.

But if you do decide to drink alcohol, drink in moderation and choose low-carb drinks like rum, vodka, tequila, whiskey and gin. The best option is dry wine and light beer.

Common Mistakes And How To Avoid Them

Choosing the wrong fasting schedule:

There are different types of IF schedules, like 16:8 (fasting for 16 hours and eating within an 8-hour window), 5:2 (eating normally for 5 days and restricting calories for 2 days), and Eat Stop Eat (fasting for 24 hours once or twice a week). Choosing the wrong one can lead to frustration and hinder results.

How to avoid it: Listen to your body and choose a schedule that fits your lifestyle and preferences. Start slow and gradually increase the fasting duration if you're a beginner.

Not eating enough during eating windows:

While IF restricts your eating window, it doesn't mean you should undereat. Aim for nutrient-dense, whole foods that keep you feeling full and satisfied. Restricting calories too much can slow down your metabolism and make it harder to lose weight in the long run.

How to avoid it: Focus on quality over quantity. Choose protein, healthy fats, and complex carbohydrates to keep you energized throughout your eating window. Listen to your hunger cues and eat until you're comfortably full, not stuffed.

Overeating during eating windows:

The freedom of an eating window can sometimes lead to overindulgence. This can negate the calorie-burning benefits of IF and hinder your progress.

How to avoid it: Practice mindful eating. Be present at your meals, chew slowly, and savor each bite. Pay attention to your hunger and fullness cues and stop eating when you're satisfied.

Not staying hydrated:

Dehydration can mimic hunger pangs and make you feel uncomfortable during your fast. It's crucial to stay hydrated throughout the day, even during fasting periods.

How to avoid it: Drink plenty of water, unsweetened tea, and black coffee throughout the day. Aim for eight glasses of water daily and adjust based on your activity level and climate.

Ignoring underlying health conditions:

If you have any underlying health conditions like diabetes, thyroid issues, or eating disorders, consult your doctor before starting IF. Some conditions might require modifications to the fasting schedule or may not be suitable for IF at all.

How to avoid it: Always prioritize your health. Listen to your doctor's advice and adjust your IF approach if necessary to ensure your safety and well-being.

Relying solely on IF for weight loss:

While IF can be a valuable tool for weight loss, it's not a magic bullet. Combining IF with a healthy diet and regular exercise is key to sustainable results.

How to avoid it: Focus on overall lifestyle changes. Eat a balanced diet, exercise regularly, and get enough sleep. These healthy habits will support your weight loss journey and improve your overall health.

Expecting overnight results:

IF is a long-term approach, not a quick fix. It takes time for your body to adjust to the fasting schedule and start burning fat efficiently.

How to avoid it: Be patient and consistent with your efforts. Celebrate small victories and focus on progress, not perfection.

Giving up too easily:

Challenges and setbacks are inevitable on any health journey. Don't get discouraged if you slip up occasionally.

How to avoid it: Remember your goals and why you started IF. Seek support from friends, family, or online communities to stay motivated.

By avoiding these common mistakes, you can maximize the benefits of intermittent fasting and achieve your health and weight loss goals.

Ways to Fast Occasionally

Intermittent fasting (IF) has garnered attention as a revolutionary approach to health and weight management. But navigating the myriad of methods can feel overwhelming. Let's delve into some popular IF regimens, empowering you to discover the perfect fit for your lifestyle and goals:

Time-restricted eating:

16/8 method: This powerhouse involves fasting for 16 hours and confining your meals to an 8-hour window. A popular strategy is skipping breakfast and dining between noon and 8 pm.

14/10 method: Slightly less intense, this method requires a 14-hour fast with a 10-hour eating window. This may be better for beginners or those who struggle with longer fasts.

12/12 method: Ideal for absolute beginners, this method involves alternating between 12-hour fasting and eating windows. You can simply extend your overnight fast by skipping breakfast or delaying dinner.

Dietary approaches:

5:2 diet: This method involves eating normally for five days and restricting your calorie intake to 500-600 on two non-consecutive days. These "fasting days" can be any combination of two days within the week.

Eat Stop Eat: This method entails a 24-hour fast once or twice a week. Choose non-consecutive days and ensure adequate hydration and calorie intake during your eating window.

Alternate-day fasting:

Full fast every other day: This method involves complete fasting (consuming only water, black coffee, or unsweetened tea) on alternate days. This is an advanced approach and requires medical supervision due to potential risks.

Modified alternate-day fasting: This involves eating 500-700 calories on fasting days, allowing for some flexibility while still reaping the benefits of extended fasting.

Breakfast

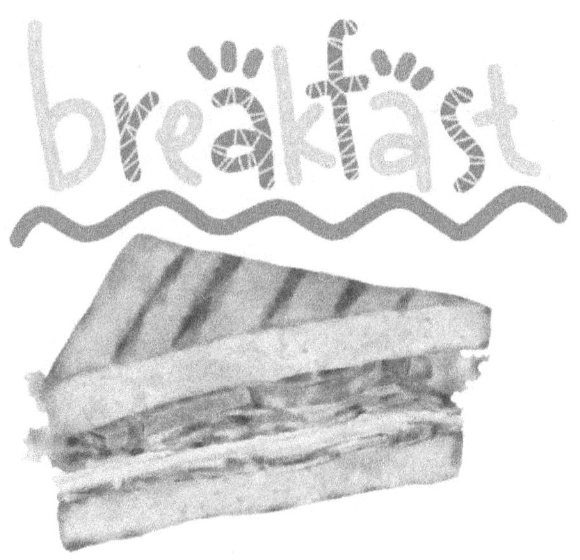

Buttery Date Pancakes

Preparation Time: 10 minutes

Cooking Time: 10 minutes Servings: 3

Nutrition: Calories: 281; Fat: 20g; Protein: 10.5g;

Carbs: 4.5g.

Ingredients:

1/4 cup almond flour 3 eggs, beaten

1 tsp. olive oil

6 dates, pitted

1 tbsp. almond butter

1 tsp. vanilla extract

1/2 tsp. ground cinnamon

Directions:

1. Stir the eggs in a bowl to make them fluffy.

2. Wash the dates and cut them in half.

3. Discard the seeds and mash them finely.

4. Melt the almond butter and add to the eggs.

5. Add the almond flour, olive oil and cinnamon.

6. Mix well and add the vanilla extract.

7. Mix into a smooth batter.

8. Add the date paste and mix well.

9. In a pan, heat the butter over medium heat.

10. Add the butter using a spoon and fry them golden brown from both sides.

11. Repeat with all the batter.

12. Serve with melted butter on top.

Chia Seed Banana Blueberry Delight

Nutrition: Calories: 260; Fat: 26.6g; Carbs: 17.4g; Protein: 4.1g.

Preparation Time: 30 minutes

Cooking Time: 0 minutes

Servings: 2

Ingredients:

1 cup yogurt

1/2 cup blueberries

1/2 tsp. Salt

1/2 tsp. Cinnamon

1 banana

1 tsp. Vanilla Extract 1/4 cup Chia Seeds

Directions:

1. Discard the skin of the banana.
2. Cut into semi-thick circles.
3. You can mash them or keep them as a whole if you like to bite into
your fruits.
4. Clean the blueberries properly and rinse well.
5. Soak the chia seeds in water for 30 minutes or longer.
6. Drain the chia seeds and transfer them into a bowl.
7. Add the yogurt and mix well.
8. Add the salt, cinnamon, and vanilla and mix again.
9. Now fold in the bananas and blueberries gently.
10. If you want to add dried fruit or nuts, add them and then serve immediately.
11. This is best served cold.

Egg Omelet

Nutrition: Calories: 289; Fat: 53.9g; Carbs: 7.9g; **Protein: 19.3g.**

Preparation Time: 10 minutes Cooking Time: 10 minutes Servings: 2

Ingredients:

1 cup cherry tomatoes 2 sausages, cooked

1 cup spinach

1/2 tsp. oregano

Salt to taste

Pepper to taste

2 eggs

2 tbsps. heavy cream

Directions:

1. Finely chop the cherry tomatoes.

2. Cut off the stem of the spinach. Chop them finely.

3. Crumble the sausage using your hands.

4. Mix the eggs with heavy cream in a bowl and add to the skillet. 5. Top the egg with cherry tomatoes, spinach, oregano and sausage. 6. Season using pepper and salt

7. Fold the omelet carefully.

8. Serve with more oregano on top.

Savory Breakfast Muffins

Nutrition: Calories: 388; Fat: 25.8g; Carbs: 8.6g; Protein: 25.3g.
Preparation Time: 10 minutes Cooking Time: 25 minutes Servings: 6
Ingredients:
8 eggs
1 cup shredded cheese
Salt and pepper to taste
1/2 tsp. baking powder
1/4 cup diced onion
2/3 cup coconut flour
11/2 cup spinach
1/4 cup full fat coconut milk

1 tbsp. basil, chopped

1/2 cup cooked chicken, diced finely

Directions:

1. Preheat the oven to 375°F.

2. Use butter or oil to grease your muffin tray or you can use muffin
paper liners.

3. In a large mixing bowl, whisk the eggs.

4. Add in the coconut milk and mix again.

5. Gradually shift in the coconut flour with baking powder and salt.

6. Add in the cooked chicken, onion, spinach, basil, and combine well.

7. Add the cheese and mix again.

8. Pour the mixture onto your muffin liners.

9. Bake for about 25 minutes.

10. Serve at room temperature.

Green Pineapple

Nutrition: Calories: 251; Fat: 0.4g; Protein: 0.5g; Carbs: 22g.

Preparation Time: 5 minutes Cooking Time: 0 minutes Servings: 3

Ingredients:

1/2 pineapple

1 broccoli, diced

1 cup water

1 long cucumber, diced A dash of salt

1 kiwi, diced

Directions:

1. Add kiwi, cucumber, pineapple, broccoli, and water in a blender.

 2. Add the salt and blend until smooth.

3. Serve.

Wholesome Mushroom and Cauliflower Risotto

Nutrition: Calories: 230; Carbs: 8g; Protein: 7.5g; Fat: 18g.

Preparation Time: 15 minutes

Cooking Time: 7 minutes

Servings: 4

Ingredients:

1 medium cauliflower head, cut into florets 1 lb. shiitake mushrooms, sliced

3 medium garlic cloves, peeled and minced 2 tbsps. coconut aminos

1 cup homemade low-sodium chicken stock 1 cup full-fat coconut milk

1 tbsp. coconut oil, melted

1 small onion, finely chopped

2 tbsps. almond flour 1/4 cup nutritional yeast

Directions:

1. On the Instant Pot, press "Sauté "and add the coconut oil.

2. Once hot, add the garlic, mushrooms, and onions. Sauté for 5 minutes

or until softened, stirring occasionally.

3. Add the remaining ingredients except for the almond flour. Cover and Cook for 2 minutes on high pressure.

4. When done, release the pressure naturally and remove the lid.

5. Sprinkle the almond flour over the risotto and stir to thicken. Serve and enjoy!

Morning Meatloaf

Nutrition: Calories: 592; Carbs: 2.5g; Protein: 11g; Fat: 49.5g.

Preparation Time: 10 minutes Cooking Time: 25 minutes Servings: 6

Ingredients:

11/2 lbs. breakfast sausage

6 large organic eggs

2 tbsps. unsweetened non-dairy milk

1 small onion, finely chopped

2 medium garlic cloves, peeled and minced 4 oz.
cream cheese, softened and cubed

1 cup shredded cheddar cheese

2 tbsps. scallions, chopped

1 cup water

Directions:

1. Add all the ingredients apart from water in a
large bowl. Stir until well combined.

2. Form the sausage mixture into a meatloaf and
wrap it with a sheet of aluminum foil. Ensure that
the meatloaf fits inside your Instant Pot. If not,
remove parts of the mixture and reserve them
for future use.

3. Once you wrap the meatloaf into a packet, add
1 cup of water and a trivet to your Instant Pot.
Put the meatloaf on the trivett's top.

4. Cover and cook for 25 minutes on high
pressure. When done, quickly release the
pressure. Carefully remove the lid.

5. Unwrap the meatloaf and check if the meatloaf
is done. Serve and enjoy!

Cinnamon and Pecan Porridge

Preparation Time: 10 minutes Cooking Time: 9 minutes
Servings: 2
Ingredients:
1 cup unsweetened coconut milk 1/4 cup almond butter
1 tbsp. coconut oil, melted
2 tbsps. whole chia seeds
2 tbsps. hemp seeds
1/4 cup pecans, chopped
1/4 cup walnuts, chopped
1/4 cup unsweetened and toasted coconut 1 tsp. cinnamon
Directions:
1. Put all the ingredients into the Instant Pot and mix.
2. Cover and cook for 9 minutes on high pressure.
3. When done, release the pressure naturally and remove the lid.

Grapefruit Yogurt Parfait

Nutrition: Calories: 103g; Fat: 4g; Fiber: 1g; Carbs: 3g; Protein: 22g.
Preparation Time: 10 minutes Cooking Time: 5 minutes Servings: 4
Ingredients:
1/2 cup amaranth
1 grapefruit, peeled, separated into segments, deseeded, chopped 3 tbsps. toasted coconut
Stevia to taste (optional)
1 cup plain, nonfat yogurt
Directions:
1. Place a pan over medium heat. Add amaranth and let it pop. It should take 3-5 minutes. Let it cool for a few minutes.
2. Add yogurt into a bowl. Add stevia and stir. Add 2 tablespoons of yogurt into each of 4 glasses.
3. Place a layer of grapefruit in each glass. Add 1 tablespoon of popped amaranth and sprinkle some coconut into the glasses.

4. Repeat steps 2-3 until all the ingredients are used up.

Creamy Mango and Banana Overnight Oats

Preparation Time: 10 minutes
Cooking Time: 0 minutes
Servings: 1
Ingredients:
Nutrition: Calories: 199; Fat: 8g; Fiber: 4g; Carbs: 9g; Protein: 4g.
For the Smoothie:
1 ripe banana
1/2 mango, peeled, cubed 1/2 tbsp. ground flaxseed 1 cup almond milk
For the Oats:
1/3 cup oats
1 small ripe banana, mashed 1/2 cup almond milk
1/2 tbsp. ground flaxseed
2 tbsps. chia seeds
Stevia or erythritol to taste

Directions:
1. Add all the smoothie ingredients into a blender and blend until smooth.
2. Pour into a tall glass.
3. To make the oats layer: Add oats, almond milk, flaxseed, chia seeds
and stevia into a bowl. Stir well and add banana. Mix until well
combined. Pour it over the smoothie in the glass.
4. Chill in the refrigerator overnight and serve.

Bacon and Eggs with Tomatoes

**Nutrition: Calories: 110; Fat: 10g; Fiber: 1g;
Carbs: 3g; Protein: 6g.
Preparation Time: 10 minutes Cooking Time: 20 minutes
Servings: 5**

Ingredients:
4 large ripe tomatoes, halved
8 rashers smoked back bacon, defatted 4 eggs
Salt to taste
Pepper to taste
1 tsp. vinegar
Directions:
1. Set up the grill to preheat. Let it preheat to high heat.
2. Place a rack on the grill pan. Line the pan with foil. Place tomatoes on the rack. Let it grill for 3 minutes. Place bacon along with the tomatoes.
3. Grill for 4 minutes until soft.
4. Meanwhile, place a large saucepan over medium-high heat. Fill the saucepan up to about 3/4 with water. Let it boil.
5. When it begins to boil, add vinegar and stir. Crack an egg into a bowl and slowly slide the egg into the boiling water. Repeat this, one at a time.
6. Cook each egg until it is soft boiled, for 2-3 minutes.

7. Meanwhile, divide the bacon and tomatoes into
2 plates.
8. Remove the eggs with a slotted spoon and
place them on the plates.
Sprinkle salt and pepper and serve.

LUNCH

Lamb Curry

Nutrition: Calories: 186; Total Fat: 7.2g; Saturated Fat: 2.5g; Cholesterol: 38mg; Sodium: 477 mg; Total Carbs: 16.3g; Dietary Fiber: 5g; Total Sugars: 5g; Protein: 14.4g. Preparation Time: 10 minutes Cooking Time: 4 hours Servings: 6

Ingredients:
2 tbsps. fresh ginger, grated
2 garlic cloves, peeled and minced 2 tsps.
cardamom
1 onion peeled and chopped
6 cloves
1 lb. lamb meat, cubed
2 tsps. cumin powder
1 tsp. garam masala
1/2 tsp. chili powder
1 tsp. turmeric
2 tsps. coriander
1 lb. spinach
14 oz. canned tomatoes

Directions:
1. In a slow cooker, mix lamb with tomatoes, spinach, ginger, garlic, onion, cardamom, cloves, cumin, garam masala, chili, turmeric, and coriander.
2. Stir well. Cover and cook on high for 4 hours.
3. Uncover the slow cooker, stir the chili, divide into bowls, and serve.

Zuppa Toscana with Cauliflower

Nutrition: Calories: 653; Carbs: 8g; Protein: 26g; Fat: 4g.

Preparation Time: 5 minutes

Cooking Time: 25 minutes

Servings: 4

Ingredients:

1 lb. ground Italian sausage

6 cups homemade low-sodium chicken stock 2 cups cauliflower florets

1 onion, finely chopped

1 cup kale, stemmed and roughly chopped

1 (14.5 oz.) can full-fat coconut milk

1/4 tsp. sea salt

1/4 tsp. freshly cracked black pepper

Directions:

1. On the Instant Pot, press "Sauté" and add the ground Italian sausage. Cook until brown, stirring occasionally and breaking up the meat with a wooden spoon.

2. Add the remaining ingredients except for the kale and coconut milk and stir until well combined.

3. Cover and cook for 10 minutes on high pressure. When done, release the pressure naturally and remove the lid. Stir in the kale and coconut milk. Cover and sit for 5 minutes or until the kale has wilted. Serve and enjoy!

Pork Carnitas

Nutrition: Calories: 170; Carbs: 2g; Protein: 4g; Fat: 8g.

Preparation Time: 20 minutes Cooking Time: 1 hour and 24 minutes Servings: 4

Ingredients:

6 medium garlic cloves, minced

2 tsps. ground cumin

1 tsp. smoked paprika

3 chipotle peppers in adobo sauce, minced 1 tsp.
dried oregano
2 bay leaves
1 cup homemade low-sodium chicken broth
Fine sea salt and freshly cracked black pepper
2 tbsps. olive oil
21/2 lbs. boneless pork shoulder, cut into 4 large
pieces

Directions:

1. Season the pork shoulder with sea salt, black
pepper, ground cumin, dried oregano, and
smoked paprika.
2. On the Instant Pot, press "Sauté" and add the
olive oil.
3. Once hot, add the pork pieces and sear for 4
minutes per side or until
brown.
4. Add the remaining ingredients inside your
Instant Pot. Cover and
cook for 80 minutes on high pressure. When
done, quickly release the
pressure and remove the lid.
5. Carefully shred the pork using 2 forks and
continue to stir until well
coated with the liquid.

6. Remove the bay leaves and adjust the seasoning if necessary. Serve and enjoy!

Cheesy Taco Skillet

Nutrition: Calories: 287; Fat: 8g; Fiber: 2g; Carbs: 12g; Protein: 28g.

Preparation Time: 10 minutes Cooking Time: 20 minutes Servings: 4

Ingredients:

1 lb. lean grass-fed ground beef

1 large yellow or white onion, finely chopped

2 medium-sized bell peppers, finely chopped

1 (12 oz.) can have diced tomatoes with green chilies

2 large zucchinis, finely chopped

2 tbsps. taco seasoning

3 cups fresh baby kale or fresh spinach

11/2 cups shredded cheddar cheese or shredded jack cheese

Directions:

1. In a large nonstick skillet, add the ground beef and cook until lightly brown. Drain the excess grease.

2. Add the chopped onions, chopped bell peppers, diced tomatoes with green chilies, zucchini, and taco seasoning. Cook for 5 minutes, stirring occasionally.

3. Add the fresh baby kale or spinach. Cook until wilted.

4. Cover with 11/2 cups of shredded cheddar cheese and cover with a lid.

5. Once the cheese has melted, serve and enjoy!

Mini Thai Lamb Salad Bites

Nutrition: Calories: 58; Fat: 2g; Fiber: 2g; Carbs: 20g; Protein: 5g.

Preparation Time: 10 minutes Cooking Time: 8 minutes Servings: 15

Ingredients:

1 large cucumber, cut into 0.39-inch-thick diagonal rounds 1/2 lb. (250 g.) lamb backstrap

3/4 cup cherry tomatoes quartered

1/3 cup fresh mint, loosely packed

1/3 cup fresh coriander, loosely packed 1/4 small red onion, finely diced

1 tsp. fish sauce

Juice 1 lime

Coconut oil

Directions:

1. Place the pan over medium heat and heat oil. Cook the lamb for 4 minutes on each side. Remove from heat and let it rest.

2. In a mixing bowl, toss the onions, tomatoes, mint, coriander, fish sauce, and lime juice.

3. Cut the lamb into thin strips and add to the salad bowl. Toss to combine.

4. Spoon the mixture on each cucumber cut. Chill and serve.

Bacon Egg and Sausage Cups

Nutrition: Calories: 100; Fat: 8g; Fiber: 2g; Carbs: 20g; Protein: 5g.

Preparation Time: 10 minutes Cooking Time: 20 minutes Servings: 8

Ingredients:

3 oz. breakfast sausages

2 slices bacon, chopped

4 large eggs

2 large green onions, chopped 1 oz. cheddar cheese, shredded 1 tbsp. coconut oil

Directions:

1. Preheat the oven to 350°F.

2. Grease your muffin pan and set it aside.
3. In a mixing bowl, beat the eggs together with the cheese. Set aside.
4. Brown the bacon in a nonstick skillet over medium heat. Add the crumbled sausage and cook until no longer pink.
5. Add the onion and cook until wilted. Remove the skillet from the heat and let it cool for 1–2 minutes.
6. Add the meat mixture to the egg mixture and beat well using a spoon.
7. Scoop mixture into the greased muffin pan and bake for 15–20 minutes or until the tops begin to brown. Remove from the pan and serve.

Smoked Salmon and Avocado Stacks

Nutrition: Calories: 106; Fat: 12g; Fiber: 2g; Carbs: 20g; Protein: 5g.

Preparation Time: 15 minutes

Cooking Time: 0 minutes

Servings: 6

Ingredients:

1/2 lb. smoked salmon, finely diced

1 ripe avocado, seed removed and diced 1 tbsp. chives, chopped

Fresh or dried dill leaves

3 tsps. fresh lemon juice

Black pepper, cracked

Directions:

1. Combine salmon, chives, and 1 tsp. of lemon juice in a small mixing bowl.

2. In another mixing bowl, toss the avocado, remaining lemon juice, and pepper.

3. Using a presentation ring, arrange the stacks on the serving plates. Arrange the avocado at the bottom and top it with the salmon mixture and gently press. Remove the mold and garnish the stack with dill leaves. Serve chilled.

Homemade Turkey Burger and Relish

Nutrition: Calories: 442; Protein: 47.86g; Fat: 21.17g; Carbs: 16.93g.

Preparation Time: 10 minutes

Cooking Time: 15 minutes

Servings: 4

Ingredients:

2 lbs. ground turkey, made into 4 patties 1 onion, finely chopped

1 red bell pepper, chopped up finely

3 cups red cabbage, chopped or shredded 1 tbsp. olive oil

1/4 cup balsamic vinegar

1/4 tsp. garlic salt

4 lettuce leaves, large if possible

Directions:

1. Take a large skillet pan and place over medium heat.

2. Add the olive oil and allow it to reach temperature.

3. Add the onion, red cabbage, and pepper to the pan and cook until
everything until softened.
4. Now add the balsamic vinegar and the garlic salt and combine
everything, letting it simmer for a few minutes until the contents have
been caramelized from the vinegar.
5. Remove the contents of the pan and set them aside to cool.
6. Take your turkey patties and season with salt and pepper.
7. Cook your patties for around 4 minutes on each side in either a pan or
under the grill.
8. Once cooked, transfer each patty onto a lettuce leaf and add some of
the relishes on top.

Butternut Squash Risotto

Nutrition: Calories: 337; Fat: 25g; Carbs: 9g; Protein: 8g.

Preparation Time: 10 minutes Cooking Time: 15 minutes Servings: 4

Ingredients:

2 tbsps. butter

2 tbsps. minced sage

1/4 tsp. black pepper, ground

1 tsp. minced rosemary

1 tsp. salt

1/2 cup dry sherry

4 cups riced cauliflower

1/2 cup butternut squash, cooked and mashed

1/2 cup Parmesan cheese, grated

1/2 cup Mascarpone cheese

1/8 tsp. grated nutmeg

1 tsp. minced garlic

Directions:

1. Melt your butter inside of a large frying pan turned to a medium level of heat.

2. Add your rosemary, your sage, and garlic. Cook this for about 1 minute or until this mixture begins to become fragrant.

3. Add in the cauliflower rice, pepper, salt, and mashed squash. Cook this for 3 minutes. You will know it is ready for the next step when cauliflower starts to soften up for you.

4. Add in your sherry and cook this for an additional 6 minutes, or until the majority of the liquid is absorbed into the rice, or when the cauliflower is much softer.

5. Stir in the Mascarpone cheese, Parmesan cheese, as well as nutmeg (grated).

6. Cook all of this on a medium heat level, being sure to stir it occasionally and do this until the cheese has melted and the risotto has gotten creamy. That will take around 4–5 minutes.

7. Taste the risotto and add more pepper and salt to season if you wish.

8. Remove your pan from the burner and garnish your risotto with more of the herbs as well as some grated parmesan.

9. Serve and enjoy

Chicken in Sweet and Sour Sauce with Corn Salad

Nutrition: Calories: 346; Protein: 56g; Fat: 45g.
Preparation Time: 10 minutes
Cooking Time: 23 minutes
Servings: 4
Ingredients:

2 cups plus 2 tbsps. unflavored low-fat yogurt 2 cups frozen mango chunks

3 tbsps. honey

1/4 cup plus 1 tbsp. apple cider vinegar

1/4 cup sultana

2 tbsps. olive oil, plus an amount to be brushed

1/4 tsp. cayenne pepper

5 dried tomatoes (not in oil)

2 small cloves garlic, finely chopped

4 cobs, peeled

8 peeled and boned chicken legs, peeled (about 700g) 6 cups mixed salad

2 medium carrots, finely sliced

Directions:

1. For the smoothie: in a blender, mix 2 cups of yogurt, 2 cups of ice, 1 cup of mango, and all the honey until the mixture becomes completely smooth. Divide into 4 glasses and refrigerate until ready to use. Rinse the blender.

2. Preheat the grill to medium-high heat. Mix the remaining cup of mango, 1/4 cup water, 1/4 cup vinegar, sultanas, olive oil, cayenne pepper, tomatoes, and garlic in a microwave bowl. Cover with a piece of clear film and cook in the microwave until the tomatoes become soft, for about 3 minutes. Leave to cool slightly and pass in a blender. Transfer to a small bowl. Leave 2 tablespoons aside to garnish, turn the chicken into the remaining mixture.

3. Put the corn on the grill, cover, and bake, turning it over if necessary, until it is burnt, about 10 minutes. Remove and keep warm.

4. Brush the grill over medium heat and brush the grills with a little oil. Turn the chicken legs into half the remaining sauce and 1/2 teaspoon of salt. Put on the grill and cook until the cooking marks appear and the internal temperature reaches 75°C on an instantaneous thermometer,

8 to 10 minutes per side. Bart and sprinkle a few times with the remaining sauce while cooking.
5. While the chicken is cooking, beat the remaining 2 tablespoons of yogurt, the 2 tablespoons of sauce set aside, the remaining spoonful of vinegar, 1 tablespoon of water, and 1/4 teaspoon of salt in a large bowl. Mix the mixed salad with the carrots. Divide chicken, corn, and salad into 4 serving dishes. Garnish the salad with the dressing set aside. Serve each plate with a mango smoothie.

Chinese Chicken Salad

Nutrition: Calories: 222; Protein: 2g; Fat: 10g; Sugar 6g.
Preparation Time: 15 minutes Cooking Time: 45 minutes Servings: 4
Ingredients:
For the Chicken Salad:

4 divided chicken breasts with skin and bones

1 tbsp. olive oil

Salt and freshly ground black pepper

500g asparagus, with the ends removed and cut into 3 parts diagonally 1 red pepper, peeled

Chinese condiment, recipe to follow

2 spring onions (both the white and the green part), sliced diagonally 1 tbsp. white sesame seeds, toasted

For Chinese Dressing:

120 ml vegetable oil

60 ml apple cider vinegar

60 ml soy sauce

11/2 tbsp. black sesame

1/2 tbsp. honey

1 clove garlic, minced

1/2 tsp. fresh peeled and grated ginger 1/2 tbsp. sesame seeds, toasted

60g peanut butter

2 tsps. salt

1/2 tsp. freshly ground black pepper

Directions:

1. For the chicken salad: Heat the oven to 180°C (or 200°C for a gas oven). Put the chicken breast

on a baking tray and rub the skin with a little olive oil. Season freely with salt and pepper.

2. Brown for 35 to 40 minutes, until the chicken is freshly cooked. Let it cool down as long as it takes to handle it. Remove the meat from the bones, remove the skin and chop the chicken into medium-sized pieces.

3. Blanch the asparagus in a pot of salted water for 3-5 minutes until tender. Soak them in water with ice to stop cooking. Drain them. Cut the peppers into strips the same size as the asparagus. In a large bowl, mix the chopped chicken, asparagus and peppers.

4. Spread the Chinese dressing on chicken and vegetables. Add the spring onions and sesame seeds, and season to taste. Serve cold or at room temperature.

5. For Chinese dressing: Mix all ingredients and set aside until use.

Dinner

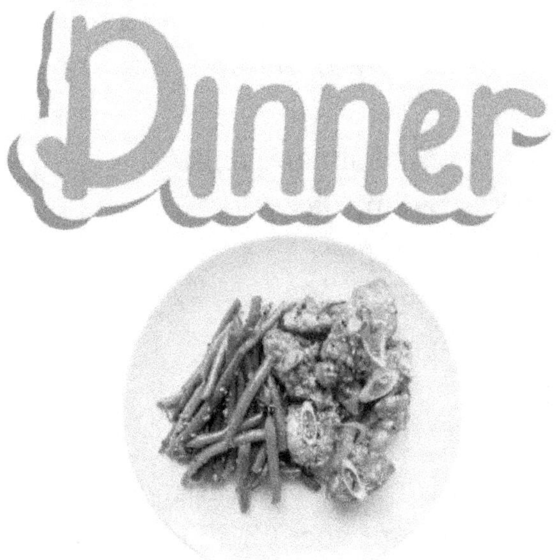

Kale & Artichoke Soup

Nutrition: Calories: 108; Fat: 8g; Fiber: 2g; Carbs: 8g; Protein: 7g.

Preparation Time: 10 minutes Cooking Time: 30 minutes Servings: 3

Ingredients:

2 cups artichoke hearts

2 cups kale leaves, tightly packed and stem discarded 32 oz. low sodium chicken broth

1/2 white sweet potato, chopped into 1/2-inch slices

1 cup unsweetened almond milk

1 large yellow onion, chopped

1 pinch cayenne pepper

1 pinch ground nutmeg

2 tbsps. Olive oil

Sea salt

Directions:

1. Place a pot over medium heat and heat the oil. Sauté the onions for about 8-10 minutes or until translucent.

2. Put in the sweet potatoes and continue to cook, stirring frequently, until soft.

3. Add the artichoke hearts, broth, nutmeg, and cayenne. Season with salt and bring to a boil.

4. Lower the heat and simmer for 10 minutes.

5. Add the kale and cover the pot with a lid. Leave it for 1 minute until

the kale leaves have wilted.

6. Add the almond milk. Next, using an immersion blender, process the mixture until smooth. Alternatively, transfer the soup to the blender and process in batches.

7. Strain the soup to separate the strands of artichoke hearts. Serve the soup hot or cold.

8. Drizzle with oil before serving.

Poached Eggs and Bacon on Toast

Nutrition: Calories: 270; Fat: 8g; Fiber: 2g; Carbs: 8g; Protein: 37g.
Preparation Time: 10 minutes
Cooking Time: 20 minutes
Servings: 1

Ingredients:

2 slices bacon

2 medium eggs

Salmon (If you want) 200g baby spinach leaves

Black pepper

Sea salt

1 slice toast

Directions:

1. Make a large pan of water to a gentle boil.

2. Stir the water gently and then break the eggs; poach for 4 minutes or
until the whites are set.

3. During that time, heat a deep frying pan, add a splash of water, and
sprinkle with the spinach. Cook for 2 minutes until the mixture is
withered.

4. Take spinach and place it aside on a plate. Fry the bacon till golden
brown.

5. Put the spinach and salmon on a toast, sprinkle with salt and pepper.

6. Cover all of it with poached eggs and bacon.

Reds Salad on Bacon and Balsamic Vinaigrette

Nutrition: Calories: 108; Fat: 50g; Fiber: 2g; Carbs: 8g; Protein: 48g.
Preparation Time: 10 minutes
Cooking Time: 10 minutes
Servings: 3
Ingredients:
1 head red leaf lettuce, torn 2 red oak leaf lettuce, torn 1/2 cup radicchio, julienned 6 streaky bacon 2 tbsps. extra virgin olive oil 1/8 cup balsamic vinegar
2 garlic cloves, grated
1 tbsp. Dijon mustard
A dash of red pepper flakes
A pinch of sea salt, add more if needed
A pinch of black pepper, add more if needed
Directions:
1. For the dressing, pour olive oil into a non-stick skillet. Fry streaky bacon for 3 minutes or until

golden brown. Transfer to a plate and crumble into small pieces. Set aside

2. In the same pan, add garlic, balsamic vinegar, Dijon mustard, red pepper flakes, salt, and pepper. Whisk until mixture is well blended. Set aside

3. To assemble, in a big salad bowl, put together red leaf lettuce, red oak leaf lettuce, and radicchio. Drizzle in dressing. Top with bacon bits. Serve.

Veggie-Stuffed Omelet

Nutrition: Calories: 150; Fat: 8g; Fiber: 2g; Carbs: 8g; Protein: 24g.

Preparation Time: 10 minutes Cooking Time: 15 minutes Servings: 1

Ingredients :

2 eggs, beaten

1/4 cup mushrooms, sliced

1 cup loosely packed contemporary baby spinach leaves, rinsed 2 tbsps. red bell pepper, chopped

1 tbsp. onion, chopped

1 tbsp. reduced-fat cheddar cheese, shredded

1 tsp. olive or canola oil

1 tbsp. water

A dash of salt

A dash of pepper

Directions :

1. Heat oil in an 8-inch non-stick skillet. Sauté the mushrooms, onion, and bell pepper for about 2 minutes until the onion is tender. Add the spinach and continue to cook, stirring frequently, until the spinach wilts. Once cooked, transfer the vegetables to a small bowl.

2. In a medium bowl, whisk the beaten eggs, water, salt, and pepper until well combined.

3. Place the same skillet in which you cooked the vegetable mixture over medium-high heat. Add the egg mixture immediately. Make a quick, sliding back-and-forth motion with the pan, using a spatula to spread the eggs at the bottom of the pan. Once the mixture is spread, let it stand for a few seconds to lightly brown the bottom of the omelet. Do not overcook it.

4. Carefully place the vegetable mixture on the half side of the omelet. Top it with cheese and, using a spatula, gently fold the other half over the vegetables. Transfer the veggie-stuffed omelet to a plate and serve.

Roasted Carrots and Cashew Salad on Lemon Vinaigrette

Nutrition: Calories: 290; Fat: 9g; Fiber: 6g; Carbs: 6g; Protein: 32g.
Preparation Time: 10 minutes
Cooking Time: 30 minutes
Servings: 2
Ingredients:
2 carrots, cubed
1/2 cup cashew nuts halved

2 tsps. cumin powder

A pinch of sea salt

A pinch of black pepper, to taste 1/2 tbsp. olive oil

1 tsp. extra virgin olive oil

1 lemon, juiced

1 tbsp. stevia

2 bags arugula, chopped

2 bags baby spinach, chopped

Directions:

1. Preheat the oven to 400°F. Line a baking sheet with parchment paper.

2. Put together olive oil, carrots, cumin powder, and cashew nuts in a
bowl. Season with salt and pepper.

3. Place mixture onto the baking sheet. Roast for 30 minutes.

4. Remove from the kitchen appliance and permit to chill for a number
of minutes.

5. To make the lemon vinaigrette, combine lemon juice, olive oil, salt,
pepper, and stevia in a separate bowl.

6. Drizzle in dressing over-cooked carrots. Set aside.

7. Put together arugula, baby spinach, and roasted veggies in a salad
bowl. Toss well to combine.
8. To serve, drizzle in just the right amount of vinaigrette over the salad.

Turmeric Tofu Scramble

Nutrition: Calories: 451; Fat: 33g; Fiber: 2g; Carbs: 8g; Protein: 21g.
Preparation Time: 10 minutes Cooking Time: 15 minutes Servings: 1
Ingredients:
1 portobello mushroom 3 or 4 cherry tomatoes
1/2 block tofu, firm
1/4 tsp. ground turmeric 1 tsp. garlic powder
Pepper and salt

1 tbsp. olive oil, some more for brushing

Directions:

1. Put the oven to a temperature of 400°F. Put the mushroom and tomatoes on a baking sheet and brush them with oil.

2. Sprinkle it with salt and pepper. Cook until tender, about 10 minutes.

3. In the meantime, mix tofu, turmeric, garlic powder, and a pinch of salt in a medium dish.

4. Mash with a fork.

5. In a large electric frying pan, over medium heat, put 1 tbsp. of olive oil. Add the tofu mixture and cook stirringly, until solid.

Raspberry Jam and Peanut Butter Overnight Oats

Nutrition: Calories: 234; Fat: 9g; Fiber: 2g; Carbs: 48g; Protein: 23g.

Preparation Time: 5 minutes

Cooking Time: 0 minutes

Servings: 2

Ingredients :

1/4 cup easy-cooking rolled oats 1/2 cup 2-percent milk

1 tsp. sugar

3 tbsps. peanut butter, creamy 3 tbsps. raspberries, (whole)

1/4 cup raspberries mashed

Directions:

1. In a medium bowl, combine oats, sugar, peanut butter, and squashed raspberries. Stir, until the batter is smooth.

2. Cover and chill overnight. In the morning, open and top with all the raspberries.

Vegan Lentil Burger

Nutrition: Calories: 560; Fat: 14g; Fiber: 2g; Carbs: 65g; Protein: 21g.

Preparation Time: 10 minutes Cooking Time: 45 minutes Servings: 6

Ingredients:

3/4 cup brown lentils

2 tsps. extra-virgin olive oil

13/4 cups low-sodium vegetable broth or water

1 large red onion, half thinly sliced and half chopped Lemon juice

Kosher salt

8 oz. fresh spinach

2 large garlic cloves, minced

Black pepper

1/2 tsp. ground cumin

1 cup whole-wheat bread crumbs

Cooking spray

1/2 cup walnuts, toasted and finely chopped

6 whole-grain vegan buns

Directions:

1. Take the lentils and 13/4 cups of the broth for boiling at high temperature in a medium saucepan. Decrease heat to medium-low, partly covered, and cook until the lentils are entirely softened, and the liquid is absorbed for around 30 minutes.

2. Mix it with the leftover 1 tablespoon of the broth and mix well with the stick blender. Set it aside.

3. Warm the oil over medium temperature in a large non-stick skillet. Add the lemon juice, chopped onion, and 1/4 teaspoon salt and cook for around 6 minutes, stirring till soft.

4. Add the spinach, garlic, 1 and a half teaspoon of black pepper and cumin, and stir until the spinach is withered for around 3 minutes.

5. Add the mixture of spinach, breadcrumbs, walnuts, and salt to the lentils and blend thoroughly. Put a cover and refrigerate for at least 1 hour or overnight.

6. Heat the grill to medium-high. Shape the mixture into 6 4-inch patties and sprinkle each side with a cooking spray. Grill till pleasant grill marks are formed, around 3 minutes per side.

Put the patties in the buns with the chopped onion and other seasonings and eat.

Vegan Coconut Kefir Banana Muffins

Nutrition: Calories: 212; Fat: 7g; Fiber: 2g; Carbs: 35g; Protein: 2g.

Preparation Time: 5 minutes

Cooking Time: 15 minutes

Servings: 6

Ingredients:

11/2 cups all-purpose flour

1 cup crushed sugar

250 ml unsweetened shredded coconut 2 tsps. baking soda

1 tsp. baking powder

1/2 tsp. salt

2 ripe mashed bananas

11/2 cups coconut milk, dairy-free
1 tsp. pure vanilla extract
1/4 cup liquid coconut oil
Directions :
1. Settle the oven to 180°C. Sprinkle cooking spray on the muffin tin. Put it aside.
2. In a big bowl, whisk together sugar, flour, baking powder, shredded coconut, salt, and baking soda. Place it aside.
3. In a separate big cup, mix together bananas, vanilla, and coconut oil. Put the flour and mix, whisk until there are no white stripes left.
4. Add the mixture to the muffin pot. Keep baking till the upper parts are golden and the spatula put in the middle comes out clean, around 30 minutes. Allow chilling the muffin tin for 15 minutes.

Chicken Tetrazzini

Nutrition: Calories: 163; Fat: 8g; Fiber: 2g; Carbs: 8g; Protein: 11g.

Preparation Time: 15 minutes Cooking Time: 25 minutes Servings: 7

Ingredients:

1/4 cup parmesan cheese, grated

1 cup mozzarella cheese, shredded

1 lb. chicken breast, boneless, skinless, & cubed 1 lb. whole wheat spaghetti noodles

1 medium onion, diced

1 tsp. oregano, dried

10 oz. button mushrooms, sliced

2 cups milk

2 medium bell peppers, diced

2 tbsps. extra virgin olive oil

3 cups chicken broth

3 large celery stalks, diced

3 tbsps. breadcrumbs

Sea salt & pepper, to taste

Directions:

1. Warm a large pot or Dutch oven over medium heat and warm the oil in it.

2. Combine celery and onion into the pot, stirring completely to combine and allowing to cook for about 3 minutes or until shiny.
3. Stir the salt, pepper, mushrooms, peppers, and oregano into the pot and stir occasionally until all ingredients get shiny and begin to cook through.
4. Stir broth, milk, parmesan cheese, and chicken into the pot and stir until completely combined.
5. Break pasta noodles in half and stir them into the mixture, doing your best to get them spread evenly throughout the pot.
6. Cover and allow to cook for about 10 minutes.
7. In a medium mixing bowl, combine mozzarella and breadcrumbs,
mixing completely.

6

8. Uncover the pot and stir once more before sprinkling the cheese and crumb mixture on top. Cover and let cook for about 3 to 5 more minutes, or until the cheese is nice and bubbly.
9. Serve hot!

Meatloaf

Nutrition: Calories: 173; Fat: 11.5g; Carbs: 0.81g; Protein: 16g.

Preparation Time: 10 Minutes Cooking Time: 40 Minutes Servings: 9

Ingredients:

2 cups, ground beef

1 cup, ground chicken

2 eggs

1 tbsp. salt

1 tsp. ground black pepper 1/2 tsp. paprika

1 tbsp. butter

1 tsp. cilantro

1 tbsp. basil

1/4 cup, fresh dill Breadcrumbs

Directions:

1. Combine chicken with ground beef in a mixing bowl.

2. Add egg, salt, ground black pepper, paprika, butter, cilantro, and basil.

3. Chop the dill and add it to the ground meat mixture and stir using your hand.

4. Place the meat mixture on aluminum foil and add breadcrumbs before
wrapping it.
5. Place it in a pressure cooker and close its lid. Cook the dish in sauté
mode and cook for 40 minutes.
6. When the cooking time ends, remove your meatloaf from the cooker
and allow it to cool.
7. Unwrap the foil, slice it, and serve.

Mixed Vegetables and Chicken Egg Rolls

Nutrition: Calories: 260; Fat: 8g; Fiber: 1g; Carbs: 8g; Protein: 23g.

Preparation Time: 10 minutes
Cooking Time: 15 minutes
Servings: 4
Ingredients:
1 tbsp. garlic, grated
1 tbsp. ginger, grated
4 tbsps. palm sugar, crumbled
1 banana chili, minced
4 tbsps. fish sauce
4 tbsps. rice wine vinegar
1 bird eye chili, minced
8 pieces spring roll wrappers Olive oil
Water, for sealing
1 garlic clove, minced
1 shallot, julienned

1/4 cup chicken, cooked shredded 1 cup bean
sprouts
1 tbsp. chicken concentrate
2 tbsps. coconut oil
1/4 cup squash, julienned
1/4 cup carrots, julienned
1/4 cup sweet potato, julienned
1/4 cup potato, julienned
1/2 cup water
A pinch of sea salt
A pinch of black pepper
Directions:
1. Combine dipping sauce ingredients in a bowl.
Stir until sugar dissolves. Taste; adjust seasoning
if needed. Set aside.
2. To make spring rolls: pour coconut oil into a
large wok set over medium heat. Sauté garlic and
shallot until limp and transparent; except for
bean sprouts, add in remaining filling
ingredients. Cook

8

until root crops are fork-tender. Toss in bean
sprouts; stir. Turn off the heat immediately. Allow

filling to cool completely to room temperature before rolling.

3. Add an equal portion of vegetable filling into spring roll paper; roll tightly, tucking in the edges and sealing with water. Set aside. Repeat step for remaining filling/wrapper.

4. Half-fill deep fryer with cooking oil set at medium heat. Cook only until spring rolls turn golden brown, about 7 minutes. Transfer cooked pieces on a plate lined with paper towels. Place 2 spring rolls on a plate; serve with dipping sauce on the side.

Soups

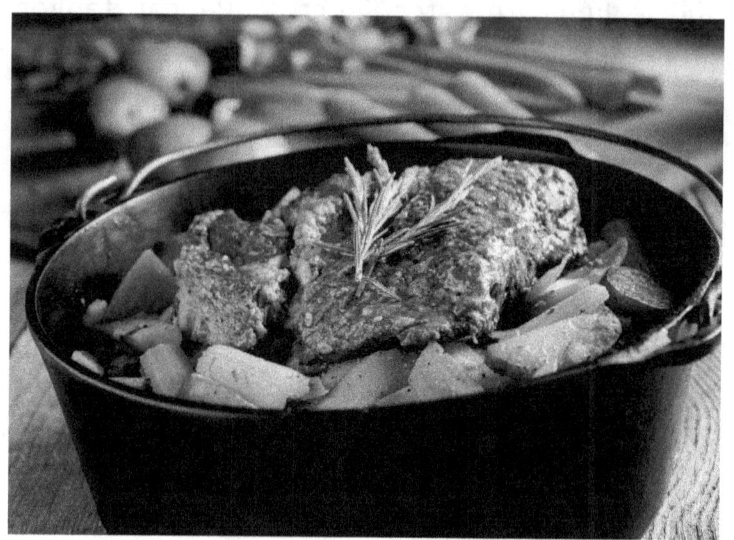

Chicken Turnip Soup

Nutrition: Calories: 186; Fat: 13.6g; Total Carbs: 3.3g; Fiber: 2.6g; Protein: 15.2g

Preparation Time: 10 minutes **Cooking Time:** 6 to 8 hours **Servings:** 5

Ingredients:

12 oz. (340g) bone-in chicken 1/4 cup turnip, chopped

1/4 cup onions, chopped

4 garlic cloves, smashed

4 cups water

3 thyme sprigs

2 bay leaves

Salt, to taste

1/4 tsp. freshly ground black pepper

Directions:

1. Put the chicken, turnip, onions, garlic, water, thyme sprigs, and bay leaves in a slow cooker.

2. Season with salt and pepper, then give the mixture a good stir.

3. Cover and cook on low for 6 to 8 hours until the chicken is cooked through.

4. When ready, remove the bay leaves and shred the chicken with a fork.

5. Divide the soup among 5 bowls and serve.

Garlicky Chicken Soup

Nutrition: Calories: 243; Fat: 22.5g; Total Carbs: 7.0g; Fiber: 6.6g; Protein: 9.6g.
Preparation Time: 10 minutes Cooking Time: 10 minutes Servings: 4
Ingredients:
2 tbsps. butter
1 large chicken breast cut into strips 4 oz. (113 g) cream cheese, cubed
2 tbsps. Garlic Gusto Seasoning
1/2 cup heavy cream
141/2 oz. (411 g) chicken broth
Salt, to taste
Directions:
1. Place a saucepan over medium heat and add butter to melt.
2. Add chicken strips and sauté for 2 minutes.
3. Add cream cheese and seasoning, and cook for 3 minutes, stirring
occasionally.

4. Pour in the heavy cream and chicken broth.
Bring the soup to a boil,
then lower the heat.
5. Allow the soup to simmer for 4 minutes, then
sprinkle with salt.
6. Let cool for 5 minutes and serve while warm.

Cauliflower Curry Soup

Nutrition: Calories: 342; Fat: 29.1g; Total Carbs: 18.3g; Fiber: 5.5g; Protein: 7.17g.
Preparation Time: 15 minutes Cooking Time: 26 minutes Servings: 4
Ingredients:
2 tbsps. avocado oil
1 white onion, chopped
4 garlic cloves, chopped

1/2 serrano pepper, seeds removed and chopped
1-inch ginger, chopped
1/4 tsp. turmeric powder
2 tsps. curry powder
1/2 tsp. black pepper
1 tsp. salt
1 cup water
1 large cauliflower, cut into florets
1 cup chicken broth
1 can unsweetened coconut milk
Cilantro, for garnish

Directions:

1. Place a saucepan over medium heat and add oil to heat.
2. Add onions to the hot oil and sauté them for 3 minutes.
3. Add garlic, Serrano pepper, and ginger, then sauté for 2 minutes.
4. Add turmeric, curry powder, black pepper, and salt. Cook for 1 minute after a gentle stir.
5. Pour water into the pan, then add cauliflower.
6. Cover this soup with a lid and cook for 10 minutes. Stir constantly.

7. Remove the soup from the heat and allow it to cool a room
temperature.
8. Transfer this soup to a blender and purée the soup until smooth.
9. Return the soup to the saucepan and add broth and coconut milk.
Cook for 10 minutes more and stir frequently.
10. Divide the soup into 4 bowls and sprinkle the cilantro on top
for garnish before serving.

Beef Taco Soup

Nutrition: Calories: 205; Fat: 13.3g; Total Carbs: 4.4g; Fiber: 0.8g; Protein: 8.0g.
Preparation Time: 15 minutes Cooking Time: 24 minutes Servings: 8
Ingredients:

2 garlic cloves, minced 1/2 cup onions, chopped 1 lb. (454 g) ground beef 1 tsp. chili powder

1 tbsp. ground cumin

1 (8 oz./227g) package cream cheese, softened

2 (10 oz./284g) cans diced tomatoes and green chilies 1/2 cup heavy cream

2 tsps. salt

2 (141/2 oz./411g) cans beef broth

Directions:

1. Take a large saucepan and place it over medium-high heat.

2. Add garlic, onions, and ground beef to the soup and sauté for 7

minutes until beef is browned.

3. Add chili powder and cumin, then cook for 2 minutes.

4. Add cream cheese and cook for 5 minutes while mashing the cream

cheese into the beef with a spoon.

5. Add diced tomatoes and green chilies, heavy cream, salt and broth

then cook for 10 minutes.

6. Mix gently and serve warm.

Creamy Tomato Soup

Nutrition: Calories: 203; Fat: 17.7g; Total Carbs: 13.0g; Fiber: 5.6g; Protein: 3.7g.
Preparation Time: 15 minutes Cooking Time: 30 minutes Servings: 4
Ingredients:

2 cups water

4 cups tomato juice

3 tomatoes, peeled, seeded and diced 14 leaves fresh basil

2 tbsps. butter

1 cup heavy whipping cream

Salt and black pepper, to taste

Directions:

1. Take a suitable cooking pot and place it over medium heat.

2. Add water, tomato juice, and tomatoes, then simmer for 30 minutes.

3. Transfer the soup to a blender, then add basil leaves.

4. Press the pulse button and blend the soup until smooth.

5. Return this tomato soup to the cooking pot
and place it over medium
heat.
6. Add butter, heavy cream, salt, and black
pepper. Cook and mix until
the butter melts.
7. Serve warm and fresh.

Chicken Soup

**Nutrition: Calories: 145; Fats: 12g; Carbs: 1g;
Protein: 8g.
Preparation Time: 25 minutes Cooking Time: 1
hour and 25 minutes Servings: 4
Ingredients:**

6 cups water

1 chicken

1 medium carrot

1 yellow onion

1 bay leaf
1 leek
2 garlic cloves
1 tbsp. dried thyme
1/2 cup white wine, dry (no, not for drinking) 1
tsp. peppercorns
Salt and pepper
Directions:
1. Peel and cut your veggies. Brown them in oil in
a big pot.
2. Split your chicken in half, down in the middle.
Pour water and spices
into the pot. Let it simmer for 1 hour.
3. Take out the chicken, save the meat, and toss
away the bones.
4. Put the meat back in the pot, and let it simmer
on medium heat for 20–
25 minutes again, while seasoning to your liking.

Roasted Butternut Squash Soup

Nutrition: Calories: 254; Fats: 15g; Carbs: 19g; Protein: 6g.

Preparation Time: 15 minutes Cooking Time: 43 minutes

Servings: 4

Ingredients:

1 large butternut squash, cubed and peeled 1 stalk celery, sliced

2 potatoes, peeled, chopped

1 onion, chopped

1 large carrot, chopped 3 tbsps. olive oil

1 tbsp. fresh thyme

25 oz. chicken broth

1 tbsp. butter Salt and pepper

Directions:

1. Preheat your oven to 400°F. On a baking sheet, toss squash and potatoes with 2 tbsps. oil and season to your taster. Roast for 20-25 minutes.

2. In the meantime, melt your butter and the rest of the oil in a large pot over medium heat. Add the onion, celery, carrot, and cook for 5-8 minutes. Season them, too.

3. Add roasted squash and potatoes. Then pour over the chicken broth. Simmer it for 10 minutes using an immersion blender until the soup is creamy.

4. Garnish it with thyme.

Cauli Soup

Nutrition: Calories: 37; Fats: 1g; Carbs: 3g; Protein: 3g.

Preparation Time: 5 minutes Cooking Time: 25 minutes Servings: 6

Ingredients:

32 oz. vegetable broth 1 head cauli, diced

2 garlic cloves, minced 1 onion, diced

1/2 tbsp. olive oil

Salt and pepper

Grated parmesan, sliced green onion for topping

Directions:

1. In a pot, heat oil over medium heat, while adding the onion and garlic. Then cook them for 4-5 minutes.

2. Add in the cauli and vegetable broth. Boil it and then cover for 15-20 minutes while covered.

3. Pour all contents of the pot into a blender and season it.

4. Blend until smooth. Top it with your cheese and green onion.

Thai Coconut Soup

Nutrition: Calories: 227; Fats: 17g; Carbs: 3g; Protein: 19g.

Preparation Time: 10 minutes Cooking Time: 35 minutes Servings: 4

Ingredients:

3 chicken breasts

9 oz. coconut milk

9 oz. chicken broth

2/3 tbsps. chili sauce

18 oz. water

2/3 tbsps. coconut aminos 2/3 oz. lime juice

2/3 tsps. ground ginger

1/4 cup red boat fish sauce Salt and pepper

Directions:

1. Slice up the chicken breasts thinly. Make them bite-sized.

2. In a large stockpot, mix your coconut milk, water, fish sauce, chili

sauce, lime juice, ginger, coconut aminos, and broth. Bring to a boil.

3. Stir in chicken pieces. Then reduce the heat and cover the pot, while
simmer for 30 minutes.
4. Remove the basil leaves and season them.

Chicken Ramen Soup

Nutrition: Calories: 478; Fats: 39g; Carbs: 3g; Protein: 31g.
Preparation Time: 10 minutes Cooking Time: 20 minutes Servings: 2
Ingredients:
1 chicken breast
2 eggs
1 zucchini, made into noodles
4 cups chicken broth
2 cloves garlic, peeled and minced 2 tbsps. coconut aminos
3 tbsps. avocado oil

1 tbsp. ginger

Directions:

1. Pan-fry the chicken in avocado oil in a pan until brown.

2. Hard boil your eggs and slice them in half.

3. Add chicken broth to a large pot and simmer with the garlic, coconut aminos, and ginger. Then add in the zucchini noodles for 4-5 minutes.

4. Put the broth into a bowl, top it with eggs and chicken slices, and season to your liking.

Creamy Tomato Soup

Nutrition: Calories: 203; Fat: 17.7g; Total Carbs: 13.0g; Fiber: 5.6g; Protein: 3.7g.

Preparation Time: 15 minutes Cooking Time: 30 minutes Servings: 4

Ingredients:

2 cups water

4 cups tomato juice

3 tomatoes, peeled, seeded and diced 14 leaves fresh basil

2 tbsps. butter

1 cup heavy whipping cream

Salt and black pepper, to taste

Directions:

1. Take a suitable cooking pot and place it over medium heat.

2. Add water, tomato juice, and tomatoes, then simmer for 30 minutes.

3. Transfer the soup to a blender, then add basil leaves.

4. Press the pulse button and blend the soup until smooth.

5. Return this tomato soup to the cooking pot and place it over medium
heat.

6. Add butter, heavy cream, salt, and black pepper. Cook and mix until
the butter melts.

7. Serve warm and fresh.

Desserts

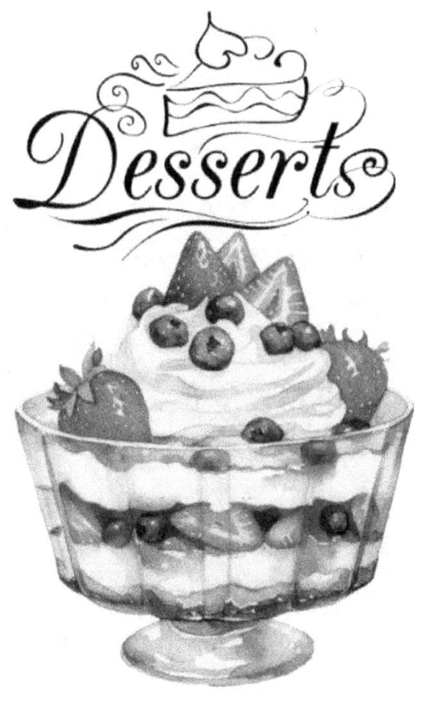

Pumpkin Ice Cream

Nutrition: Calories: 293; Total Fat: 22.5g; Saturated Fat: 20.1g; Cholesterol: 0mg; Sodium: 99mg; Total Carbs: 24.8g; Fiber: 3.6g; Sugar: 14.1g; Protein: 2.3g.

Preparation Time: 15 minutes Cooking Time: 0 minutes Servings: 6

Ingredients:

15 oz. homemade pumpkin puree

1/2 cup dates, pitted and chopped

2 (14-oz) cans of unsweetened coconut milk 1/2 tsp. organic vanilla extract

11/2 tsp. pumpkin pie spice

1/2 tsp. ground cinnamon

A pinch of sea salt

Directions:

1. In a high-speed blender, add all the ingredients and pulse until smooth.

2. Transfer into an airtight container and freeze for about 1-2 hours.
3. Now, transfer the mixture into an ice cream maker and process it
according to the manufacturer's directions.
4. Return the ice cream to the airtight container and freeze for about 1-2
hours before serving.

Avocado Pudding

Nutrition: Calories: 462; Total Fat: 20.1g; Saturated Fat: 4.4g; Cholesterol: 0mg; Sodium: 13mg; Total Carbs: 48.2g; Fiber: 10.2g; Sugar 30.4g; Protein: 3g.
Preparation Time: 15 minutes Cooking Time: 0 minutes Servings: 4
Ingredients:
2 cups bananas, peeled and chopped
2 ripe avocados, peeled, pitted, and chopped 1 tsp. fresh lime zest, grated finely

1 tsp. fresh lemon zest, grated finely

1/2 cup fresh lime juice

1/2 cup fresh lemon juice

1/3 cup agave nectar

Directions:

1. In a blender, add all the ingredients and pulse until smooth.

2. Transfer the mousse into 4 serving glasses and refrigerate to chill for
about 3 hours before serving.

Chocolate Mousse

Nutrition: Calories: 357; Total Fat: 13g; Saturated Fat: 1.7g; Cholesterol: 0mg; Sodium: 26mg; Total Carbs: 52.1g; Fiber: 11.9g; Sugar: 16.7g; Protein: 13.4g.

Preparation Time: 10 minutes Cooking Time: 0 minutes Servings: 4

Ingredients:

1/2 cup unsweetened almond milk

1 cup cooked black beans

4 Medjool dates, pitted and chopped 1/2 cup pecans, chopped

2 tbsps. non-alkalized cocoa powder 1 tsp. organic vanilla extract

4 tbsps. fresh blueberries

Directions:

1. In a food processor, add all the ingredients and pulse until smooth and creamy.

2. Transfer the mixture into serving bowls and refrigerate to chill before serving.

3. Garnish with blueberries and serve.

Apple Crisp

Nutrition: Calories: 100; Total Fat: 2.7g; Saturated Fat: 0.8g; Cholesterol: 0mg; Sodium: 3mg; Total Carbs: 19.1g; Fiber: 2.6g; Sugar: 11.9g; Protein: 1.2g.

Preparation Time: 15 minutes Cooking Time: 20 minutes Servings: 8

Ingredients:

For Filling:

2 large apples, peeled, cored, and chopped 2 tbsps. water

2 tbsps. fresh apple juice

1/4 tsp. ground cinnamon

For Topping:

1/2 cup quick rolled oats

1/4 cup unsweetened coconut flakes 2 tbsps. pecans, chopped

1/2 tsp. ground cinnamon

1/4 cup water

Directions:

1. Preheat the oven to 300oF. Lightly grease a baking dish.
2. To make the filling add all of the ingredients to a large bowl and
gently mix. Set this aside.
3. Make the topping by adding all of the ingredients to another bowl and
mix well.
4. Place the filling mixture into the prepared baking dish then spread the
topping over the filling mixture evenly.
5. Bake for about 20 minutes or until the top becomes golden brown.
6. Serve warm.

Chocolate Crunch Bars

Nutrition: Calories: 316; Total Fat: 30.9g; Saturated Fat: 8.1g; Cholesterol: 0mg; Total Carbs: 8.3g; Sugar: 1.8g; Fiber: 3.8g; Sodium: 8mg; Protein: 6.4g.

Preparation Time: 5 minutes Cooking Time: 3 minutes Servings: 4

Ingredients:

11/2 cups sugar-free chocolate chips 1 cup almond butter

Stevia to taste

1/4 cup coconut oil

3 cups pecans, chopped

Directions:

1. Layer an 8-inch baking pan with parchment paper.

2. Mix chocolate chips with butter, coconut oil, and sweetener in a bowl. 3. Melt it by heating in a microwave for 2 to 3 minutes until well mixed. 4. Stir in nuts and seeds. Mix gently.

5. Pour this batter into the baking pan and spread evenly.

6. Refrigerate for 2 to 3 hours.

7. Slice and serve.

Homemade Protein Bar

Nutrition: Calories: 179; Total Fat: 15.7g; Saturated Fat: 8g; Cholesterol: 0mg; Total Carbs: 4.8g; Sugar: 3.6g; Fiber: 0.8g; Sodium: 43mg; Protein: 5.6g.

Preparation Time: 5 minutes Cooking Time: 0 minutes Servings: 4

Ingredients:

1 cup nut butter

4 tbsps. coconut oil

2 scoops vanilla protein Stevia, to taste

1/2 tsp. sea salt

1 tsp. cinnamon (Optional)

Directions:

1. Mix coconut oil with butter, protein, stevia, and salt in a dish. 2. Stir in cinnamon and chocolate chips.

3. Press the mixture firmly and freeze until firm.

4. Cut the crust into small bars.

5. Serve and enjoy.

Shortbread Cookies

Nutrition: Calories: 288; Total Fat: 25.3g; Saturated Fat: 6.7g; Cholesterol: 23mg; Total Carbs: 9.6g; Sugar: 0.1g; Fiber: 3.8g; Sodium: 74mg; Potassium: 3mg; Protein: 7.6g.

Preparation Time: 10 minutes Cooking Time: 15 minutes Servings: 6

Ingredients:

21/2 cups almond flour 6 tbsps. nut butter

1/2 cup erythritol

1 tsp. vanilla essence

Directions:

1. Preheat your oven to 350°F.

2. Layer a cookie sheet with parchment paper.

3. Beat butter with erythritol until fluffy.

4. Stir in vanilla essence and almond flour. Mix well until becomes

crumbly.

5. Spoon out a tablespoon of cookie dough onto the cookie sheet.

6. Add more dough to make as many cookies.

7. Bake for 15 minutes until brown.

8. Serve.

Peanut Butter Bars

Nutrition: Calories: 214; Total Fat: 19g; Saturated Fat: 5.8g; Cholesterol: 15mg; Total Carbs: 6.5g; Sugar: 1.9g; Fiber: 2.1g; Sodium: 123mg; Protein: 6.5g.
Preparation Time: 10 minutes Cooking Time: 0 minutes Servings: 6
Ingredients:
3/4 cup almond flour 2 oz. almond butter 1/4 cup Swerve
1/2 cup peanut butter 1/2 tsp. vanilla
Directions:
1. Combine all the ingredients for bars.
2. Transfer this mixture to a 6-inch small pan. Press it firmly. 3. Refrigerate for 30 minutes.
4. Slice and serve.

Zucchini Bread Pancakes

Nutrition: Calories: 246; Carbs: 49.2g; Fiber: 4.6g; Protein: 7.8g.

Preparation Time: 15 minutes Cooking Time: 8 minutes Servings: 3

Ingredients:

1 tbsp. grapeseed oil

1/2 cup chopped walnuts

2 cups walnut milk

1 cup shredded zucchini

1/4 cup mashed burro banana 2 tbsps. date sugar

2 cup kamut flour or spelled

Directions:

1. Place the date sugar and flour into a bowl. Whisk together.

2. Add in the mashed banana and walnut milk. Stir until combined. Remember to scrape the bowl to get all the dry mixture. Add in walnuts and zucchini. Stir well until combined.

3. Place the grapeseed oil onto a griddle and warm.

4. Pour 1/4 cup batter on the hot griddle. Leave it along until bubbles
begin forming on the surface. Carefully turn over the pancake and cook
for another 4 minutes until cooked through.
5. Place the pancakes onto a serving plate and enjoy with some agave
syrup.

Berry Sorbet

Nutrition: Calories: 99; Carbs: 8g; Fiber: 6.7g; Protein: 12.8g
Preparation Time: 10 minutes Cooking Time: 10 minutes Servings: 6
Ingredients:
2 cups water
2 cups blend strawberries 11/2 tsp. spelled flour
1/2 cup date sugar
Directions:
1. Pour the water into a large pot and let the
water begin to warm. Add the flour and date

sugar and stir until dissolved. Allow this mixture to start boiling and continue to cook for around 10 minutes. It should have started to thicken. Take off heat and set to the side to cool.

2. Once the syrup has cooled off, add in the strawberries, and stir well to combine.

3. Pour into a container that is freezer safe and put it into the freezer until frozen.

4. Take sorbet out of the freezer, cut into chunks, and put it either into a blender or a food processor. Hit the pulse button until the mixture is creamy.

5. Pour this into the same freezer-safe container and put it back into the freezer for 4 hours.

Quinoa Porridge

Nutrition: Calories: 180; Fat: 3g; Carbs: 40g; Protein: 10g.

Preparation Time: 5 minutes Cooking Time: 15 minutes Servings: 4

Ingredients:

Zest 1 lime

1/2 cup coconut milk 1/2 tsp. cloves

11/2 tsp. ground ginger 2 cup spring water

1 cup quinoa

1 grated apple

Directions:

1. Cook the quinoa according to the instructions on the package. When the quinoa has been cooked, drain well. Put it back into the pot and stir in spices.

2. Add coconut milk and stir well to combine.

3. Grate the apple now and stir well.

4. Divide equally into bowls and add the lime zest on top. Sprinkle with

nuts and seeds of choice.

Apple Quinoa

Nutrition: Calories: 146; Fiber: 2.3g; Fat: 8.3g; Carbs: 15.6g; Protein: 1.5g.

Preparation Time: 15 minutes Cooking Time: 15 minutes Servings: 4

Ingredients:

1 tbsp. coconut oil Ginger

1/2 key lime

1 apple

1/2 cup quinoa

Optional Toppings:

Seeds Nuts Berries

Directions:

1. Fix the quinoa according to the instructions on the package. When you are getting close to the end of the cooking time, grate in the apple and cook for 30 seconds.

2. Zest the lime into the quinoa and squeeze the juice in. Stir in the coconut oil.
3. Divide evenly into bowls and sprinkle with some ginger.
4. You can add in some berries, nuts, and seeds right before you eat.

Kamut Porridge

Nutrition: Calories: 114; Protein: 5g; Carbs: 24g; Fiber: 4g.
Preparation Time: 10 minutes Cooking Time: 25 minutes Servings: 4
Ingredients:
4 tbsps. agave syrup 1 tbsp. coconut oil 1/2 tsp. sea salt
1 cup coconut milk 1 cup kamut berries
Optional Toppings:
Berries Coconut chips Ground nutmeg Ground cloves

Directions:

1. You need to "crack" the Kamut berries. You can do this by placing the berries into a food processor and pulsing until you have 11/4 cups of Kamut.

2. Put the cracked Kamut in a pot with salt and coconut milk. Give it a good stir to combine everything. Allow this mixture to come to a full rolling boil and then turn the heat down until the mixture is simmering. Stir every now and then until the Kamut has thickened to your likeness. This normally takes about 10 minutes.

3. Take off heat, stir in agave syrup and coconut oil.

4. Garnish with toppings of choice and enjoy.

Blueberry Cupcakes

Nutrition: Calories: 85; Fat: 0.7g; Carbs: 12g; Protein: 1.4g; Fiber: 5g.

Preparation Time: 15 minutes Cooking Time: 30 minutes Servings: 4

Ingredients:

Grapeseed oil

1/2 tsp. sea salt

1/4 cup sea moss gel 1/3 cup agave

1/2 cup blueberries 3/4 cup teff flour

3/4 cup spelled flour 1 cup coconut milk

Directions:

1. Heat your oven to 365o. Place paper liners into a muffin tin.

2. Place sea moss gel, sea salt, agave, flour, and milk in a large bowl.
Mix well to combine. Gently fold in blueberries.

3. Gently pour batter into paper liners. Place in oven and bake for 30 minutes.

4. They are done when they have turned a nice golden color, and they
spring back when you touch them.

Snack

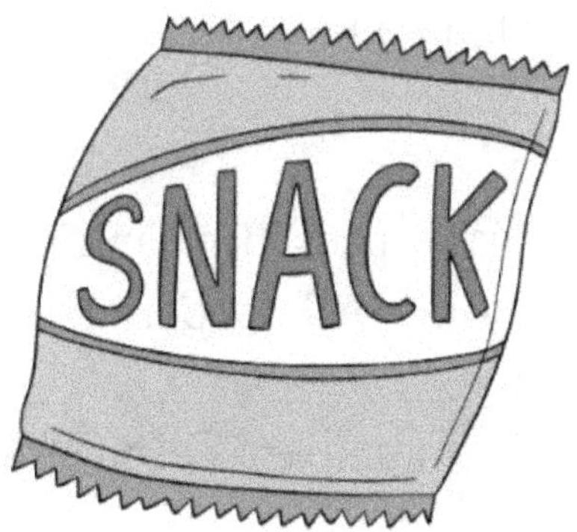

Pepperoni Bites

Nutrition: Calories: 59; Fat: 4.5g; Fiber: 0.1g;
Carbs: 2g; Protein: 2.5g.

Preparation Time: 5 minutes Cooking Time: 10 minutes Servings: 24 pieces

Ingredients:

1/3 cup tomatoes, chopped

1/2 cup bell peppers, mixed and chopped 24 pepperoni slices

1/2 cup tomato sauce

4 oz. almond cheese, cubed

2 tbsps. basil, chopped

Black pepper to taste

Directions:

1. Divide pepperoni slices into a muffin tray.

2. Divide tomato and bell pepper pieces into the pepperoni cups.

3. Also divide the tomato sauce, basil, and almond cheese cubes,

sprinkle black pepper at the end, place cups in the oven at 400°F, and

bake for 10 minutes.

4. Arrange the pepperoni bites on a platter and serve.

5. Enjoy!

Party Meatballs

Nutrition: Calories: 71; Fat: 2.6g; Fiber: 2.2g; Carbs: 4.1g; Protein: 7.7g.

Preparation Time: 10 minutes Cooking Time: 8 minutes Servings: 20

Ingredients:

1 lb. turkey meat, ground 1 tbsp. coconut oil, melted 1 yellow onion, chopped 1 egg

1 cup coconut flour

1 tsp. Italian seasoning

A pinch sea salt

Black pepper to taste

2 tbsps. parsley, chopped

Directions:

1. In a bowl, mix turkey meat with half of the flour, a pinch of salt, black pepper, Italian seasoning, parsley, onion, egg, and hot sauce and stir well.

2. Put the rest of the flour in another bowl.

3. Shape 20 turkey meatballs and dip each 1 in flour.

4. Heat up a pan with the oil over medium-high heat, add meatballs,
cook them for 4 minutes on each side, transfer to paper towels to
remove any excess grease, place all of them on a platter and serve.
5. Enjoy!

Artichoke Petals Bites

Nutrition: Calories: 93; Protein: 6.54g; Fat: 3.72g; Carbs: 9.08g.
Preparation Time: 10 minutes Cooking Time: 10 minutes Servings: 8
Ingredients:
8 oz. artichoke petals, boiled, drained, without salt 1/2 cup almond flour
4 oz. parmesan, grated
2 tbsps. almond butter, melted
Directions:
1. In the mixing bowl, mix up together almond flour and grated Parmesan.

2. Preheat the oven to 355°F.
3. Dip the artichoke petals in the almond butter and then coat in the
almond flour mixture.
4. Place them in the tray.
5. Transfer the tray to the preheated oven and cook the petals for 10
minutes.
6. Chill the cooked petal bites a little before serving.

Stuffed Beef Loin in Sticky Sauce

Nutrition: Calories: 321; Protein: 18.35g; Fat: 26.68g; Carbs: 2.75g.
Preparation Time: 15 minutes
Cooking Time: 40 minutes
Servings: 4

Ingredients:

1 tbsp. erythritol

1 tbsp. lemon juice

1 tbsp. butter

1/2 tsp. tomato sauce

1/4 tsp. dried rosemary

9 oz. beef loin

3 oz. celery root, grated 3 oz. bacon, sliced

1 tbsp. walnuts, chopped 3/4 tsp. garlic, diced

2 tsps. butter

1 tbsp. olive oil

1 tsp. salt

1/2 cup water

Directions:

1. Cut the beef loin into the layer and spread it with the dried rosemary, butter, and salt. Then place over the beef loin: grated celery root, sliced bacon, walnuts, and diced garlic.

2. Roll the beef loin and brush it with olive oil. Secure the meat with the help of the toothpicks. Place it in the tray and add a 1/2 cup of water.

3. Cook the meat in the preheated to 365°F oven for 40 minutes.

4. Meanwhile, make the sticky sauce: Mix up together Erythritol, lemon

juice, 4 tablespoons of water, and butter.
5. Preheat the mixture until it starts to boil. Then add tomato sauce and
whisk it well.
6. Bring the sauce to boil and remove from the heat.
7. When the beef loin is cooked, remove it from the oven and brush it
with the cooked sticky sauce very generously.
8. Slice the beef roll and sprinkle with the remaining sauce.

Almond Flour Muffins

Nutrition: Calories: 75; Carbs: 4g; Fat: 6g; Protein: 0g.
Preparation Time: 15 minutes Cooking Time: 30 minutes Servings: 8
Ingredients:
1/3 cup pumpkin puree 3 eggs
2 tbsps. agave nectar 2 tbsps. coconut oil

1 tsp. vanilla extract 1 tsp. white vinegar 1 cup chopped fruits 1 tsp. baking soda 1/2 tsp. salt

Directions:

1. Preheat the oven to 350°F.
2. Line the muffin tin with paper liners
3. In the first mixing bowl, whisk the almond flour, salt, and baking soda.
4. In the second mixing bowl, whisk the pumpkin puree, eggs, coconut oil, agave nectar, vanilla extract, and vinegar.
5. Now add this puree mix of the second bowl to the first bowl and blend everything well.
6. Add the chopped fruits to the blend.
7. Pour the mixture into the muffin cups in your pan.
8. Bake for 15-20 minutes. Ensure that the contents have been set in the center, and a golden-brown lining has started to appear at the edges.
9. Transfer the muffins to a cooling rack and let them cool completely.

Eggplant Fries

Nutrition: Calories: 212; Fat: 15.8g; Carbs: 12.1g; Protein: 8.6g

Preparation Time: 10 minutes Cooking Time: 15 minutes Servings: 8

Ingredients:

2 eggs

2 cups almond flour

2 tbsps. coconut oil, spray

2 eggplant, peeled and cut thinly Salt and pepper

Directions:

1. Preheat your oven to 400°F.

2. Take a bowl and mix with salt and black pepper in it

3. Take another bowl and beat eggs until frothy

4. Dip the eggplant pieces into eggs

5. Then coat them with a flour mixture

6. Add another layer of flour and egg

7. Then, take a baking sheet and grease it with coconut oil on top 8. Bake for about 15 minutes

9. Serve and enjoy.

Roasted Broccoli

Nutrition: Calories: 62, Fat: 4g;
Carbs: 4g; Protein: 4g.
Preparation Time: 5 minutes Cooking Time: 20
minutes Servings: 4
Ingredients:
4 cups broccoli florets 1 tbsp. olive oil
Salt and pepper to taste
Directions:
1. Preheat your oven to 400°F
2. Add broccoli in a zip bag alongside oil and shake until coated 3. Add seasoning and shake again
4. Spread broccoli out on the baking sheet, bake for 20 minutes 5. Let it cool and serve.

30 Days Meal Plan

Here are three more examples of different fasting time windows you can choose from, each with its own benefits and considerations:

The Early Bird Special: 6 am - 2 pm

This shorter fasting window, known as the 18/6 method, is perfect for early risers who like to fuel their mornings with a delicious breakfast.

Benefits:

- May be easier to maintain for beginners who find longer fasts challenging.
- Promotes early calorie burning and increased energy throughout the day.
- Provides ample time for a nutritious and satisfying lunch before the fasting window begins.

Considerations:

- May require an adjustment to your sleep schedule if you're not used to waking up early.
- May not be suitable for individuals with social engagements or late-night commitments.

The Midday Warrior: 10 am - 6 pm no

This 16/8 method is an excellent option for individuals who prefer a later breakfast or who find themselves naturally fasting in the morning.

Benefits:

- Allows for flexibility in scheduling your meals and snacks within the eating window.
- Aligns with natural circadian rhythms,potentially improving sleep quality.
- May be easier to manage for those with active lifestyles or busy mornings.

Considerations:

- May require skipping dinner or having a light meal later in the evening.
- May not be suitable for individuals who work late or have evening social commitments.

The Night Owl's Delight: 2 pm - 10 pm

This 20/4 method, also known as the OMAD (One Meal a Day) approach, involves condensing your daily calorie intake into a single eating window.

Benefits:

- May offer the most significant metabolic benefits in terms of fat burning and insulin sensitivity.
- Provides maximum flexibility throughout the day and can be incorporated into various lifestyles.
- May promote improved digestion and gut health.

Considerations:

- Requires careful planning and portion control to ensure adequate nutrient intake within the single eating window.
- May not be suitable for individuals with certain health conditions or those who struggle with hunger pangs.
- Can be socially isolating, especially during dinner gatherings.

Remember, the best fasting time is the one that fits your lifestyle and preferences. Experiment with different options and find what works best for you.

Days	Breakfast	Lunch	Dinner	Dessert
1	Avocado Egg Bowls	Smoked Salmon and Avocado Stacks	Maple Walnut-Glazed Black-Eyed Peas with Collard Greens	Chocolate Mousse
2	Low Carb Pancake Crepes	Homemade Turkey Burger and Relish	Reds Salad on Bacon and Balsamic Vinaigrette	Shortbread Cookies
3	Awesome Oatmeal	Chinese Chicken Salad	Savory Oatmeal Bowl	Chocolate Crunch Bars
4	Cinnamon Porridge	Creamy Lamb Korma	Instant Pot Teriyaki Chicken	Homemade Protein Bar
5	Creamy Mango and Banana Overnight Oats	Butter Chicken	Peanut Butter Bars	Roasted Broccoli with Lemon, Garlic and Toasted Pine Nuts
6	Cinnamon and Pecan Porridge	Zuppa Toscana with Cauliflower	Roasted Carrots and Cashew Salad on Lemon Vinaigrette	Zucchini Bread Pancakes
7	Egg Omelet	Pork Carnitas	Vegan Lentil Burger	Brazil Nut Cheese
8	Chia Seed Banana Blueberry Delight	Bacon Egg and Sausage Cups	Chicken Tetrazzini	Baked Apples
9	Savory Breakfast Muffins	Asparagus and Pistachios Vinaigrette	Mixed Vegetables and Chicken Egg Rolls	Pumpkin Ice Cream

10	Morning Meatloaf	Pork Carnitas	Turmeric Tofu Scramble	Apple Quinoa
11	Sesame- Seared Salmon	Teriyaki Salmon	Poached Eggs and Bacon on Toast	Blueberry Cupcakes
12	Eggs and Salsa	Butternut Squash Risotto	Quick and Easy Squash Soup	Kamut Porridge
13	Grapefruit Yogurt Parfait	Mini Thai Lamb Salad Bites	Meatloaf	Overnight "Oats"
14	Keto Oatmeal	Garlic Butter Beef Steak	Veggie- Stuffed Omelet	Apple Crisp
15	Poached Egg	Instant Pot Teriyaki Chicken	Kale & Artichoke Soup	Apple Quinoa
16	Wholesome Mushroom and Cauliflower Risotto	Sesame- Seared Salmon	Vegan Coconut Kefir Banana Muffins	Avocado Pudding
17	Green Pineapple	Cheesy Taco Skillet	Filipino Chicken Adobo	Berry Sorbet
18	Savory Breakfast Muffins	Asparagus and Pistachios Vinaigrette	Mixed Vegetables and Chicken Egg Rolls	Pumpkin Ice Cream
19	Bacon and Eggs with Tomatoes	Lamb Curry	Asparagus and Green Peas Salad	Chocolate Crunch Bars
20	Low Carb Pancake Crepes	Homemade Turkey Burger and Relish	Instant Pot Teriyaki Chicken	Berry Sorbet
21	Cinnamon and Pecan Porridge	Salmon with Sauce	Sesame- Ginger Chicken Salad	Baked Apples

22	Cinnamon Porridge	Lamb Curry	Vegan Coconut Kefir Banana Muffins	Shortbread Cookies
23	Savory Breakfast Muffins	Cheesy Taco Skillet	Meatloaf	Brazil Nut Cheese
24	Avocado Egg Bowls	Garlic Butter Beef Steak	Asparagus and Green Peas Salad	Blueberry Cupcakes
25	Awesome Oatmeal	Butter Chicken	vegan Lentil Burgers	Quinoa Porridge
26	Sesame- Seared Salmon	Zuppa Toscana with Cauliflower	Maple Walnut-Glazed Black-Eyed Peas with Collard Greens	Homemade Protein Bar
27	Cinnamon and Pecan Porridge	Bacon Egg and Sausage Cups	Reds Salad on Bacon and Balsamic Vinaigrette	Peanut Butter Bars
28	Buttery Date Pancakes	Smoked Salmon and Avocado Stacks	Savory Oatmeal Bowl	Chocolate Mousse
29	Eggs and Salsa	Sesame- Seared Salmon	Filipino Chicken Adobo	Overnight "Oats"
30	Grapefruit Yogurt Parfait	Mini Thai Lamb Salad Bites	Roasted Carrots and Cashew Salad on Lemon Vinaigrette	Zucchini Bread Pancakes

CONCLUSION

You've reached the final page of this journey, and somewhere along the way, you likely shed more than just pounds. You shed doubt, you shed limitations, and you shed years off your body and spirit. Remember, age is just a number, but the way you choose to move through it, the fire you ignite within, that's what truly defines you.

As Dr. Mark Mattson, renowned neuroscientist, states, "Age is not destiny. We can influence how we age through lifestyle choices." You've made one of the most powerful choices, embracing intermittent fasting and unlocking a new wave of energy and well-being.

But remember, this isn't the end, it's the beginning. Carry the principles of IF into your daily life, fueling your body with nourishment, challenging yourself with movement, and most importantly, celebrating every victory, big or small.

As Deepak Chopra reminds us, "The greatest glory in living lies not in never falling, but in rising every time we fall." There will be stumbles, temptations, and setbacks, but within you lies the resilience to overcome them. Keep your gaze on the horizon, on the vibrant, healthy future you've built.

Finally, carry the torch of inspiration. Share your success, your knowledge, and your enthusiasm with others. As Dr. Michael Mosley, creator of the 5:2 diet, proclaims, "The best time to start intermittent fasting was six months ago. The second best time is now." Be the catalyst for change in someone else's life, just as this book has been for you.